FAT

Reference Point

FAT

SHERRY ASHWORTH

Cover illustration by
David Scutt

Inside illustrations by
Polly Dunbar

SCHOLASTIC

Scholastic Children's Books,
Commonwealth House, 1-19 New Oxford Street
London WC1A 1NU, UK
a division of Scholastic Ltd
London ~ New York ~ Toronto ~ Sydney ~ Auckland

First published in the UK by Scholastic Ltd, 1997

ISBN 0 590 19012 1

Typeset by TW Typesetting, Midsomer Norton, Avon
Printed by Cox and Wyman Ltd, Reading, Berks

10 9 8 7 6 5 4 3 2 1

Contents

Chapter 1

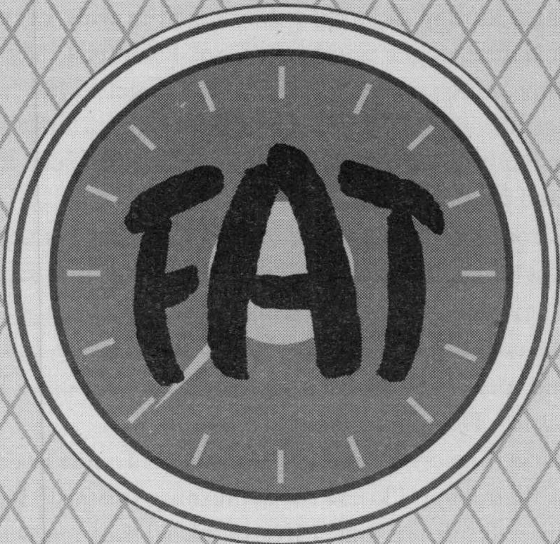

The 'F' word

Theresa is 15, and has a problem…

Dear Sue,

I know I'm not thin – I'm bigger than normal, I think. Not that it used to bother me very much. My figure's not what I want it to be, but I can't say it's on my mind all the time. Then one Saturday morning I'd arranged to walk over to my friend's house to get a video – Cool Runnings. My friend lives a few streets away from me, and to get to her house, I had to go through a cul-de-sac, and through a little alley. I was in a really good mood. It was a hot day, I'd seen the film before and it was brilliant.

Then from the other side of the road, these boys appeared. I knew who they were, although they weren't friends of mine. They went to another school. I was wearing jeans and a skinny rib jumper. So now there were these four boys following me. One of them said, very loudly, 'Look! There's that fat girl!' Then all of them laughed.

Of course, I ignored them, and walked on. To retaliate is to go down to their level. I knew I was blushing furiously but I just hoped they didn't see that. I felt awful. Half of me wanted to bash them – I was in such a rage – but I felt humiliated too, like I wanted to go and hide in a cupboard. I choked back the tears. It's an absolutely horrible feeling, having someone call you fat. It sends your self-esteem plummeting to rock-bottom. I wouldn't have minded if they had said, look at her hair – she's dyed it bright pink. People who look different deliberately have the character to take the flak. Being called 'fat' is another thing entirely, because you can't help the way you are.

When I got to my friend's house I told her what had happened and she said the boys were being pathetic. I know they were, but it doesn't change my feelings. All that day, whenever I looked in the mirror, I thought I looked horrible, and I could see why the boys said I was fat. My friend said to me that since my dress size was only 12, I couldn't possibly be fat. But my thighs are massive. I knew those boys wouldn't have called me fat if there wasn't a reason. There's no smoke without fire.

I enjoyed the video, but I couldn't help thinking, should I do something about being fat? I wondered about dieting – so many of my friends won't eat chocolate now, and some of them even skip school lunch. On the one hand, I know it's the person inside that counts, but more than anything I don't want those boys to call me fat again. So if I was slimmer, maybe they wouldn't.

Yours,
Theresa

Dear Theresa,

Your friend is right. The boys in question were pathetic – they were only trying to wind you up. You're not fat, and even if you were, you have the right to make decisions about the size you want to be. You don't have a problem: the boys who called you fat have a problem – with the size of their brains. All you need to do is learn to be happy with the shape you are. Your personality is far more important than your appearance, and from your account, you sound a sensitive and thoughtful girl. So forget all about the unkind comments, and get a life!

Sue Slim, Agony Aunt

But is it that easy to forget all about your weight? What would happen if Theresa had a chance to answer back to Sue?

Stop – I can't stand it! You sound just like my mum! It's all very well to say that personality is more important than your appearance, but people's first impressions of you are based on your appearance. Boys in the street don't call out, 'Look at her personality!' And anyway, it's AWFUL being fat.

Theresa

Who are you?

Sue

I'm Theresa, alias Miss Blobby. That's what my mirror tells me. And when I turn around and look at myself sideways on, it's worse. My thighs have wobbly bits and my stomach sticks out. Last night I tried lying on the floor with an encyclopaedia on my tummy, but it didn't work. I just don't want to be fat.

But you're not fat.

How can you say that? I'm covered in fat.

So is everyone. We need our fat – it stores energy, keeps us warm, and would even save our lives if we were marooned halfway up a mountain.

That's great, except I don't go mountaineering. My fat's useless, unless I wanted to get a job as a circus freak.

Aren't we guilty of a little exaggeration here? You seem pretty normal to me. Just because you can grab a handful of flesh at the top of your thighs doesn't mean you're fat. Stomachs are designed to stick out, especially after meals. Don't confuse yourself with your old Barbie doll.

All right, forget my stomach and thighs for a moment. I know I'm fat because the scales say so. I've put on weight recently. Don't tell me it's normal to keep putting weight on.

It is if you're growing taller. Are you sure your bathroom scales are accurate? If they're nearly as old as your parents, it's likely they'll be inaccurate. Not only that, but you can even have a different weight at different times of the day. You weigh less if you're dehydrated, more if you're constipated, less if it's first thing in the morning, more if you're expecting a period, more if you stand on the scales forgetting that you're holding the cat.

But you've got to keep a check on your weight!

Says who? Weighing yourself every day doesn't make you slimmer – it just makes you obsessed with your weight. You don't keep measuring yourself every day to see if you're growing taller, do you?

At least the scales are kinder than the mirror. When I look in the mirror, it's like Frankenstein's monster is let loose in my bedroom.

Do you have one of those distorting mirrors in your bedroom? Like the sort you get in the hall of mirrors in fairgrounds?

No. It's an ordinary one. And it tells the truth. I'm fat.

Are your eyes telling the truth? I bet when you look in the mirror you've already decided what you're going to see when you look there. If you stare at your stomach, it seems bigger, because whatever you focus on grows and fills your whole vision. And if you look in the mirror believing that you're gross, you'll make yourself find the evidence to prove it. If you look in the mirror thinking you're sex on two legs, then you *will* be sex on two legs. How we look in the mirror determines what we see. Do you smile when you look in the mirror? Or do you twist your eyes and rotate you shoulder like the Hunchback of Notre Dame so you can focus on the spot on the left-hand corner of your chin? If you do, you'll look like the Hunchback of Notre Dame.

So if I can't trust the scales or my mirror, who can I trust? My mum tells me I'm not fat, but that's only because she loves me. My friends won't tell me if I'm fat, because they don't want to hurt my feelings.

So let me get this right: the people who care for you are the last people on earth you'd trust. Logic isn't really your strong point, is it?

Who says being fat is a logical issue? I FEEL fat!

So you've admitted it. Fat is an emotional issue. Perhaps what you've got covering your body isn't real fat so much as mental fat.

What's mental fat?

That dimply, revolting stuff that you can see all over your body, which is invisible to everybody else. We all have it. It's called mental fat because it only exists in your mind, and when you go on about how fat you are, you'll drive yourself and your friends mental. You don't get mental fat from too many chocolate biscuits, but from thinking about fat too much, and you don't need to diet to get rid of it. You just have to stop believing in it. Then it goes.

I wish. But I know I'm fat because everybody around me is slimmer than me. You know, at school. You look around and everyone looks thinner than you.

To you they do. But again, you might be distorting what you see with your own prejudices about yourself. You might be looking around your friends picking out the people who are slimmer than you. And even if you are slightly bigger than some girls, does anyone else notice? Even if you're half a stone heavier than the girl sitting next to you, it won't be visible to the naked eye, and it won't even be visible if you're both naked. The problem's in your head, not on your body.

But I was called fat even though you say I'm not fat. I reckon fat is the real 'F' word.

You're too right. One of the reasons you go on about being fat, is that 'fat' is used as a term of abuse. 'Fatty' is a playground insult in primary school, and it's one that the teachers don't often pick up on, because they don't see anything wrong with it, as it seems petty to them. Yet try calling a teacher fat, and see what happens!

When you come to think about it, it's strange that it's rude to call someone fat. Why should it be?

First of all, that's not true everywhere in the world. In some countries, fleshy women are desirable – the more, the better! Sadly, in Western society, fatness has always been ridiculed. Children read Billy Bunter books, seaside postcards poke fun at fat people, and reactions to them range from pity through amusement to dislike. Psychologists and sociologists and all the other '-gists' will come up with hundreds of reasons why this is so. Whatever the reasons, the problem remains. It doesn't feel good to be called fat.

Isn't that because fat people are greedy, and it's wrong to be greedy? I've read the Billy Bunter books, and he's always stuffing himself. There's a girl in my class who's bigger than me, and she has a Mars bar every break.

Is she the only one? Do the rest of you have lettuce leaves and cottage cheese for break, then?

No, we have Mars bars too.

81 per cent of the world's cultures think plumpness or moderate fatness is desirable for females.

So you're all greedy. Or perhaps it's normal to want some chocolate after a hard morning solving chemical equations. Why should only slim people eat chocolate? That doesn't sound fair to me.

But I thought you had to eat a lot to get fat.

Not always. There can be medical reasons why people suffer from obesity. Then some people can't help overeating in the way some alcoholics find it impossible to stop drinking. Very, very few people actually want to be fat, but they might find it difficult to lose weight. Some people eat loads, but never put weight on. To look at a fat person and assume they're eating too much is judging by appearances, and judging only by appearances is prejudice.

So laughing at fat people is like being racist. I'd never make jokes about fat people, anyway.

But you've been making jokes about yourself. Fat prejudice is a funny thing because people who've got it don't just hate others, but give themselves a hard time. Check you're not prejudiced against yourself.

You're making my head spin. But I agree with you, really. It's wrong to call people fat. I think we ought to ban the word 'fat'. From now on, I'm going to call fat people, large, or plump, or cuddly.

But surely if being fat is nothing to be ashamed of, we can refer quite normally to fat people, like we talk about tall people, or blondes, or redheads?

Trust you to be awkward! What I mean is, the word 'fat' has upset so many people, we shouldn't say it ever again.

Some fat people might prefer the honest description 'fat'. If you call an overweight person 'cuddly' she might think you were too embarrassed to talk about her as she really is, or that you were patronizing her.

I know! Here's an even better idea. Everyone should use the word 'fat' for good things, instead of 'cool' or 'brilliant'. Here goes. 'I've had a fat holiday'. Or, 'My dad gave me double pocket money this week, which is really fat.' Or, 'Do you want to go to see a film with me? Yeah, fat!' Then it won't matter if we call people fat.

Now that's a fat idea…

QUIZ

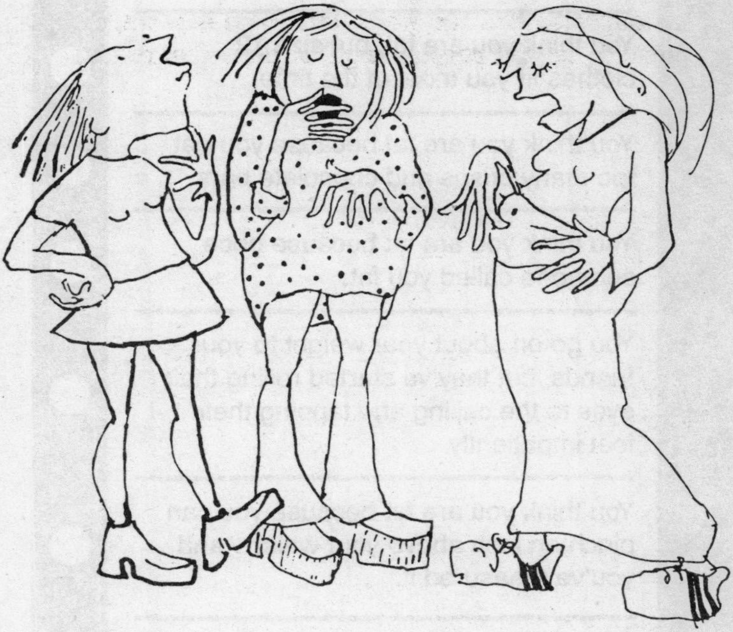

If you think you are fat, answer the following questions. For each statement you can tick, you are awarded two points.

Do you suffer from mental fat?

1. You think you are fat, but your parents tell you that you're slim. ◯

You look even fatter when you are changing for games, or when you put on your school uniform.

You think you are fat, but size 12 clothes fit you most of the time.

You think you are fat because you eat too many crisps and chocolate bars.

You think you are fat because once someone called you fat.

You go on about your weight to your friends, but they've started rolling their eyes to the ceiling and tapping their feet impatiently.

You think you are fat because you can pinch an inch above your waist – and you've measured it.

You think you are fat because you look nothing like the girls of your age on TV.

You think you are fat because the clothes you wore last year no longer fit you.

You think you are fat because your mother thinks she is fat and you take after her.

How did you score?

14-20

Virtually all of your fat is mental fat. Take a good, long look at yourself. Most teenagers would kill to look like you. Don't ruin your life unnecessarily. You really have nothing to worry about.

8-12

You do tend to worry about your weight more than you need to. Check you don't become obsessed with how you look. Enjoy everything you eat – even the treats.

0-6

Well done! Worrying just a little bit about your weight is normal, but you seem to keep a sense of proportion.

Chapter 2

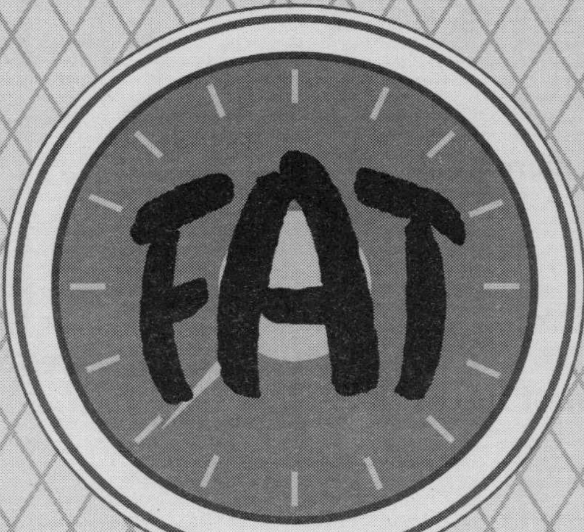

Don't let the critics grind you down!

...OK, so I've got 20lbs of mental fat. But what I want to know is, where did it all come from? If it wasn't through overeating, how come I've ended up with it...?

Imagine you had a choice. Would you buy in to adolescence?

Good morning, miss.

Good morning.

You look like a discerning sort of customer to me. Just the sort of girl who might be interested in our latest special offer.

What's that?

Would you like to be able to transform yourself into a beautiful, desirable, fully-mature young woman – all entirely free of charge?

Sounds good to me.

Then you want Adolescence! Just sit back, and let Adolescence take control of your body. In just a few years we can guarantee you'll be adult, attractive to the opposite sex, able, eventually, to have children of your own. If you'll just sign here...

Wait a minute, wait a minute. What about the small print? For example, are there any unpleasant side-effects?

Ahem! Well, obviously, as your body develops there are changes which might – ahem!

Out with it. I want to know the downside of adolescence too.

Very quickly, then, they are:

growth of hair underneath arms and in pubic area

monthly loss of blood from genitalia

necessity to ask adult for tampons or sanitary towels

spots

changes in appearance of genitalia

growth of breasts, which might bounce as you run

necessity to be measured for your correct bra size

putting on of weight in hip area

dramatic mood swings from elation to depression

greasy hair

painful crushes on boys who don't know you exist

Omigod! How EMBARRASSING! I don't think I'll bother, thank you ... excuse me...

Not so fast, young lady. Adolescence isn't optional. It happens to us all, and it's happening to you.

Aaargh!

Growing up makes us feel self-conscious. First, there's our embarrassment about the changes themselves. It's awful to be the first girl in your class to have to wear a bra, and just as awful to be the last. It's awful to need a bra, and your mother refuses to buy you one. You also look silly if you wear a bra and you don't need one. Growing breasts is a minefield of embarrassment.

Worse are the changes in your genital area. The books tell you to expect hair, but when it grows it's wiry and rough. And the books might not have told you that the skin around the opening to your vagina grows too. So don't worry, you're not deformed.

Noticing all these changes is bad enough, but adolescence also brings with it feelings of embarrassment, of self-consciousness, sometimes even a feeling of self-disgust. You watch your body growing and changing and think 'Yeeeeuch!!!'

And it's hard to put this feeling into words, so you say instead, 'I'm fat'. Just at a time in your life when you want people not to notice you, your body is absolutely intent on being noticed. It's excruciatingly embarrassing. You wish you could grow smaller; your body's growing bigger. No wonder you wish to control it.

Myth . . . Myth . . . Myth . . . Myth . . . Myth

It's only puppy fat, dear. You'll soon lose it when you're a teenager.

But there's no such thing as puppy fat. On reaching adolescence, you GAIN weight. Your body needs to lay down deposits of fat on your hips and on your breasts to help you feed babies when or if you eventually decide to have them. Women and teenage girls are supposed to go out and in and out.

Here's what some girls had to say about themselves:

'I hate my hips and bum – they're huge. My bum sticks out at the back!'
(Alice, 15)

'I hate the tops of my arms and my legs. They're all fleshy.'
(Natalie, 13)

'I hate my thighs and tummy. My tummy's not flat – it kind of sticks out.'
(Sharon, 13)

'I hate my thighs – they're massive!'
(Christine, 14)

Alice, Natalie and Sharon all wear dress size 10; Christine is size 12.

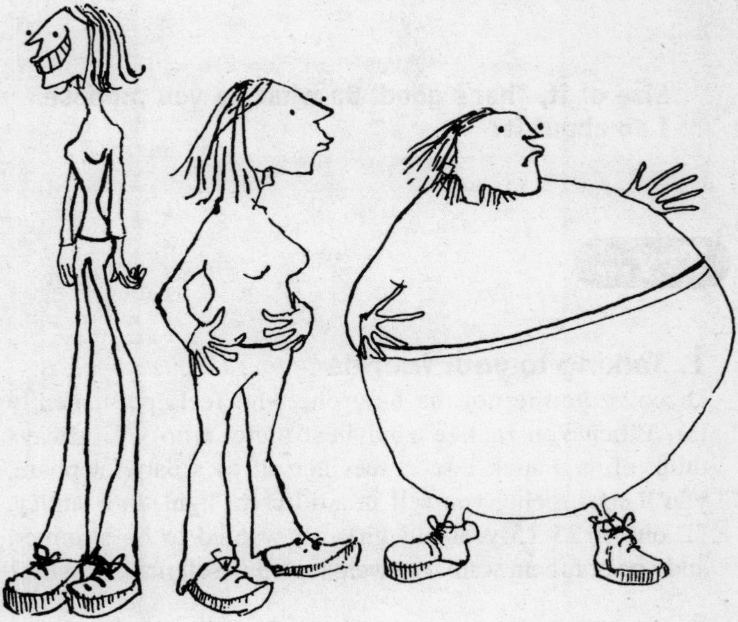

What girls think they ought to look like.

What a normal teenage girl looks like.

What she thinks she

So wait a minute. You're saying that all the changes in adolescence make me self-conscious and negative about my body, and I start hating all the bits that I think of as fat?

That's just about the size of it.

Size of it. That's good. So what do you propose I do about it?

Try...

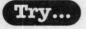

1. Talking to your friends

Discover you're not the only one who feels permanently fat. When you realize your best mate, who you always think of as a stick insect, sees herself as a baby elephant, you'll start seeing yourself in a different light. In a survey, 22 out of 25 15-year-old girls all wanted to be slimmer, and none of them were overweight. Are we all mad, or what?

2. Giving your body credit

Sit down tonight and make a list of all the things you like your body for. You might like your eyes, your hair, your skin, your feet; you might have long, elegant fingers, strong nails; you might be a good swimmer, basketball player, dancer. You might enjoy walking, aerobics, tennis. Just think: the last time you were ill, your body got better all by itself. Think how some mornings, when you wake up, you're full of energy. Write down all the compliments you've had. Make yourself believe them. This is *you*! Now stick this list on your mirror, and when you're feeling negative, read it.

3. Looking at real women

Go down to your local swimming baths, and as you're changing, or swimming lengths, have a look at the variety of shapes and sizes that other girls and women come in. I wouldn't recommend including men in your survey, as they might get the wrong idea. But you'll see that no two women or girls are identical in shape. Some women have small breasts and big hips. Others have substantial thighs but tiny hips. Others have generous busts and thick waists. The permutations are endless. Each one of us is designed to be unique. And remember, *all* thighs are flabby, *all* stomachs stick out, and *all* bums stick out too.

That's all very well. But it's like, you do all that, and you tell yourself you're all right really, and you might believe it for a day or two, and then somebody says something, and you're back to hating yourself.

You're right. Another thing about adolescence is that you don't have a strong sense of your own identity yet, so you rely very heavily on the opinions of others about you. And everybody seems to think they have the right to tell you stuff about yourself...

6/10. I like the ideas in your story but your spelling leaves a lot to be desired...

You're so messy. You never tidy your bedroom...

You're 5'2" and weigh 8 stones...

You're Gemini, so there are two distinct sides to your personality...

You've got no taste in music. That group can't play to save their lives...

Those jeans don't suit you...

I like your hair but I think the hairdresser should have left it a little longer...

Don't answer back! You're cheeky!

You are a pleasant, helpful girl, hard-working and willing to make the best of yourself...

What with school reports, parents' comments, friends, relations, brothers, sisters, teachers, doctors, we have no end of information on which to develop a view of ourselves. So what sort of comments do we listen to most? The negative ones, of course!
For most of us, the fear of not getting it right, of not fitting in, of being seen to be different, means that we react much more strongly to criticism than to praise.

My brother's 18. We get on most of the time, and now he's away at university it's not so bad. But you should see him. He's dead skinny, and he can eat whatever he likes. So he sits there, and just comes out with comments: don't eat that Mars bar – you'll get fat. Or he'll say, here's my fat sister, Nellie the elephant. Or he'll call me thunder thighs. I know he's only teasing, and I suppose if I was really fat, he wouldn't call me fat. But on the other hand, why would he call me fat if there was no reason? So I end up believing him, and not believing him. Whichever, it still hurts. I've told him to stop but he doesn't see a problem with it. He thinks it's funny that I worry about my weight all the time – to him it's just a big joke.
(Eleanor, 16)

At school, when you're in the fifth year, they give you a medical. Well, I suppose they have to. But what I don't like is that the doctor weighs you. And then she has this chart, and she tells you whether you're normal or not. She told me I was slightly overweight. I was devastated. When you come out of her office, all your friends say, how much do you weigh? Or they try to sneak a look at your card. It's horrible. ***(Mandy, 15)***

This is what I can't stand. You're getting changed for games or swimming and there are these girls – always the dead skinny ones – who pinch the skin around their waist and go 'Ooh! aren't I fat? It's so disgusting. I'm going to have to go on a diet.' Then you look at yourself and you see all your rolls of fat, and you think, well, if she's going on a diet, I'm going to have to starve myself. I'm much fatter than her. Or your friend looks around the changing room, and points out a really thin girl, and says, I wish I had legs like hers. And you look at your legs and see how much fatter they are. Everybody's so competitive. ***(Anna, 14)***

My aunt – the one I go to after school until my mum gets home – it's not that she's ever said to me that I'm fat or anything. But it's, 'You'd better not have any biscuits. Have an apple instead; it's healthier.' And sometimes she looks at me, and says, 'You look as if you've lost weight. Well done.' She said that once after I'd had a tummy bug and didn't eat all weekend. I thought, you're mad, you – I've been ill. But also at the same time I was very pleased, and I thought I'd try not to eat too much for the rest of the week, so I wouldn't put that weight back on. My aunt's dead figure conscious and goes to aerobics three times a week. ***(Kylie, 14)***

It was lunchtime in school and I was sitting on the desk with my mates. Now we're not supposed to do that, sit on the desks. I don't know why because the teachers do. So I'm sitting there, in my school uniform skirt that I'd rolled up, to make it shorter, chatting, and the teacher on duty comes in. Before I could slide off the desk she goes, 'Off the desk, Pat. It's an ugly sight, that vast expanse of flesh.' She could see my thighs, you see. I went bright scarlet, and I thought – you cow! I mean, she wasn't exactly Kate Moss. But I couldn't say anything, could I? And all day long I felt horrible.
(Pat, 16)

Other people's comments do have a stronger effect on us than our own ideas about ourselves. Even if you know your sister calls you 'fat' to rile you, half of you believes her.

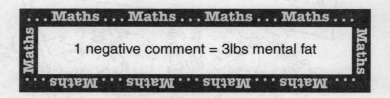

. . . Maths . . . Maths . . . Maths . . . Maths . . .

1 negative comment = 3lbs mental fat

Next time someone upsets you with an unwanted remark about your appearance, try waving this Bill of Rights at them.

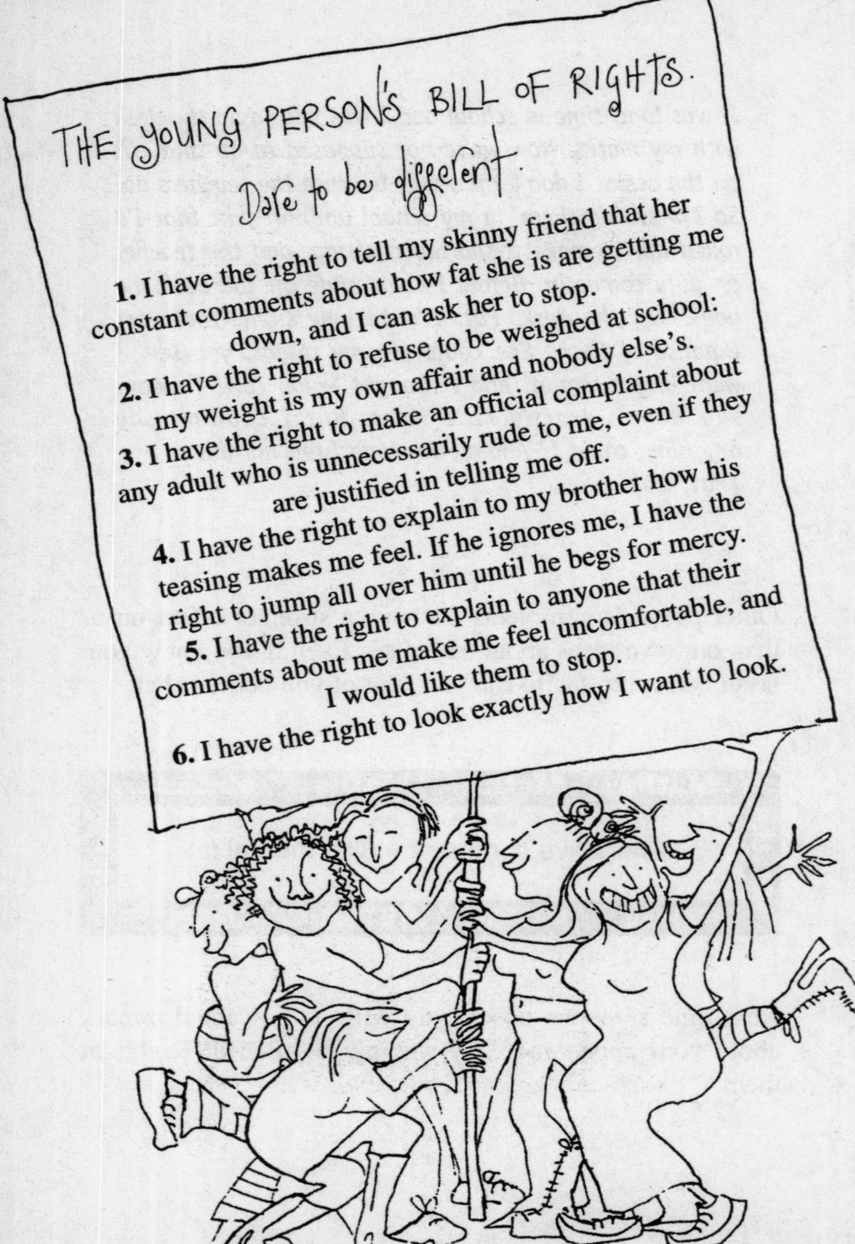
THE YOUNG PERSON'S BILL OF RIGHTS.
Dare to be different.
1. I have the right to tell my skinny friend that her constant comments about how fat she is are getting me down, and I can ask her to stop.
2. I have the right to refuse to be weighed at school: my weight is my own affair and nobody else's.
3. I have the right to make an official complaint about any adult who is unnecessarily rude to me, even if they are justified in telling me off.
4. I have the right to explain to my brother how his teasing makes me feel. If he ignores me, I have the right to jump all over him until he begs for mercy.
5. I have the right to explain to anyone that their comments about me make me feel uncomfortable, and I would like them to stop.
6. I have the right to look exactly how I want to look.

Chapter 3

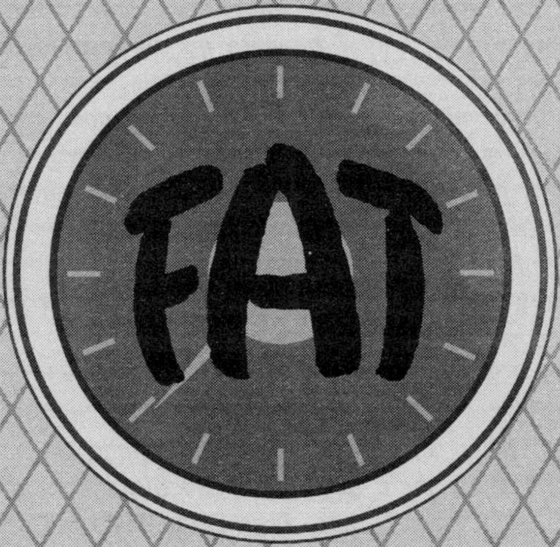

Family fortunes

Mum's the word

'Me? I like Blur and Oasis, or anything headbang-y. I love reading, literature, that sort of thing – not the sciences. And my politics are left of centre. Not like my mum! She's right wing, and she'll only listen to classical music and she can't stand my clothes. She should talk. She's so untidy, and I have to go around tidying up after her.

Yes, I see myself as fat. I'm a size 16 now, although it's true I'm tall for my age. I don't like the way I eat. I eat junk food a lot of the time – I have chocolate and things like that when I'm miserable, and then I hate myself. I don't binge or anything, but I think I should eat more healthily. Most of the time I do, but there are the odd occasions...

When I was little, it was my grandmother who picked me up from school. That was because my mother worked. When she could, my mother came to pick me up, and then she'd buy me a chocolate bar, a Curly Wurly, as a special treat. That Curly Wurly was a sign she'd thought about me. She'd have to go and buy it specially. And on family occasions, too, there'd always be lots of sweets and chocolates – it was a way of celebrating, or there'd be a cake if I'd done well at school.

Most of the time I did do well at school. I was the clever one of the family – my cousin was the good-looking one. She lost a lot of weight in her teens, and kept it off, and people were always making comments about how well Christine had done in controlling her weight, in front of me, as if I should take note. I did. It made me feel awful. Even now it makes me feel like, if I tried a little harder, I could be like her, and I hate myself sometimes for being the way I am. I can understand the appeal of dieting, even if my common sense tells me dieting doesn't work.

My mum loves cooking, and preparing food, and being with food, and she picks while she's in the kitchen, and then she won't sit down and eat with the rest of us. I know if she's upset, she'll reach for some cake. She's always complaining about her weight. She sees eating as a problem – it's a problem if you're hungry, it's like you're giving in to something. If she's too busy to have lunch she's pleased, she'll boast about it to me and the rest of us. But she buys loads of food, and then she won't eat it in case she gets fat. She goes on diets, of a sort. I know when she eats out, she'll never have a first course – that's her way of cutting down. She doesn't like to be seen eating in public. Once she bought loads of Slimfast, and was going to try that, but in the end she didn't drink them because she's a doctor, and she knows meal substitutes aren't good for you. But I suppose she was desperate. I'll tell you a funny thing she does – she eats standing up. She thinks that doesn't count.

I do understand why she's like she is. Her mother came from a very poor family, and it was only when my mum was a very little girl, that my grandmother had enough money to feed her properly. So food became a symbol of success. My grandmother was proud to be able to provide really big meals. And it was a case of 'Now I've made it, you've got to eat it. Don't waste food. Other people are starving.' My grandmother knew what it was like to starve. She used to cook for me and my mother when I was small, so I've experienced all this at first hand.

But then, when my mother was a teenager, it was different. My grandmother was very influenced by her friends, who were saying that it was important for a girl to be slim in order to get a husband. My mother was slim right up until she was 20 or so, but then she put on weight. Mr grandmother was worried, so she would encourage my mum to eat less, and lose weight. It was like a double message. Eat this meal I've made for you, but now I want you to lose weight!

I remember a big family dinner a few years ago when my grandmother was doing the cooking. She'd spent ages on this meal, and she was encouraging me to eat as much as I could. Even though I wasn't hungry, she was like, 'Eat the dessert, Helen. Go on – I made it specially.' So I did. Then after the meal, she was saying to me, 'I can't believe how much you've eaten. Why don't you lose some weight like your cousin?'

My mother isn't so obvious, but she also gives me double messages. If she sees me snacking, it's 'Don't eat so much rubbish – you know chocolate isn't good for you.' Or sometimes she'll even say, 'If you'd eaten properly at lunchtime, you wouldn't want to be filling your stomach with rubbish now.' Or she'll make a really heavy meal, and then say that she shouldn't have made that for me. My mother knows that one or two of my friends have suffered from anorexia, and she often tells me how glad she is that I'm not like that. At those times she encourages me to eat. But then she'll go shopping and fill the fridge with vegetables and cottage cheese for both of us.

It's worse if we go out shopping for clothes. If she sees that I'm fitting a size 16, she says, 'I was never that big at your age. You really ought to lose some weight.' But that same night, she might see me when

I've dressed up to go out, and she'll tell me how lovely I look, and she means it. Then there are other times, when she sees me in new clothes, and says, 'That's nice, that makes you look slim.' I can see why. My uncle – her brother – is always making jokes about fat women, particularly a neighbour of his, so I reckon she thinks it's safer to be slim, and also, of course, that you won't get a man if you're not slim. Well, that didn't apply to Dawn French!

The thing is, I love my mother more than anyone in the world. She's brilliant. She's a really strong, committed woman, she's been tremendously successful in her career, she works for good causes. I suppose people in our area know me as her daughter, rather than me in my own right. So I suppose that's why I rebel, and listen to Blur rather than Beethoven, and why I won't diet...
(Helen, 16)

Love 'er or loathe 'er, your mother is probably the biggest influence on the way you feel about yourself, and particularly the way you feel about your weight. Even if you argue with mum most of the time, or if you get on well, or even if you ignore her, or if she seems to ignore you, she's the adult female you grew up with, and unconsciously you model yourself on her.

No ... no... That can't be true!

Sorry, but it is. Ask any psychologist. She'll explain that your mum is the one female role model who's been with you since birth, and so you believe, deeply and unconsciously, that when you are fully grown, you'll be like her. For some of us, this is quite a reassuring thought. It might make the rest of us want to scream. So most teenagers are caught between trying to be like mum, and trying not to be like mum. Because once you reach your teens, you want to establish your own identity, your own look, your own habits, and you might find yourself in conflict with mum. Or you might find yourself not wanting to break away from being her little girl. The permutations are endless.

What's your mum like?

To find out what habits and ideas you might have had handed down from your mum, fill out this questionnaire, and analyse your mother. Use the prompts to help you answer the questions, but feel free to add anything else about your mother that comes to mind. Remember, just as you're unique, your mother is unique too. If you haven't lived with your mother for a long time, do the questionnaire about your closest female carer.

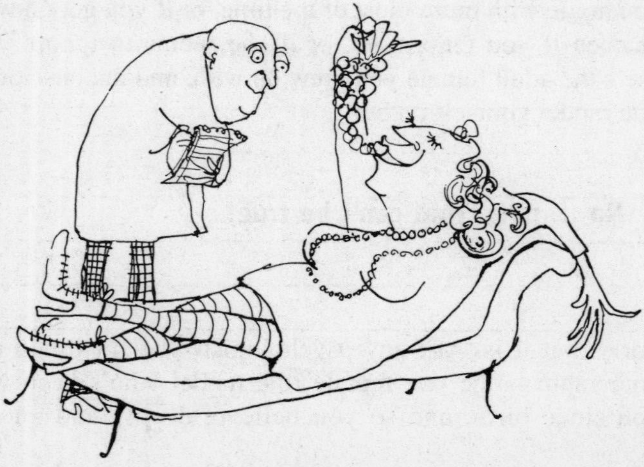

1. Describe your mother's body shape. Does she keep her body that way by constant dieting, restricting her food intake, or very frequent exercise? If she has sisters or brothers, are they a similar size to her?

2. Open your fridge and food cupboard, if your mother is the main person responsible for buying the food. (Remember, even if your dad does the shopping it might be your mum's list he's working from.) Now take a good look at the type of food around. Are there lots of treats, like biscuits, cakes, crisps? Or are there lots of diet products, low-fat spreads, diet cola, reduced sugar jams? Is there a lot of food? Or is there just enough to see you through the next day or so? Describe what you see.

3. Think of mealtimes in your house. Do you have regular mealtimes, or do people grab something when they're hungry? Now think of your mum eating. Does she eat big meals and say how much she enjoys them? Does she care more about whether you've eaten everything? Does your mother start eating while she's preparing a meal, because she's hungry? Does she eat the same as the rest of you, or differently, because she's on a diet? After the meal, does she say, 'I shouldn't have eaten that'?

4. Look carefully at your mother's appearance. Does she always wear make-up? Fashionable clothes? Does she make an effort to look young for her age? Does she often ask you what you think she looks like? Does she like to think she can still fit into the dress size she was before she had you?

5. Listen to your mother. Does she complain about being

fat? Does she talk sympathetically or critically about other women who are overweight? Does she use the word 'naughty' or 'wicked' if she eats something high in calories like chocolate, a cream cake or a rich dessert? Does she talk about dieting a lot, or tell you how she's got no willpower?

6. Now think about what your mother says to you. Does she tell you you've got to eat healthily? Does she buy lots of fruit and vegetables for you and nag you to eat them? Does she pull a face or pass a comment when she sees you eating something high in calories? Does she worry you a lot about whether you're eating enough, because she doesn't want you to get an eating disorder? Does she ask you every day what you've had for school dinner? Has she ever suggested to you that you should go on a diet/eat more healthily with her? Or has she asked or told you to diet, or to do something about your weight?

Vairy eenteresting! Just taking time to think about your mother, and her habits, might have given you some new insights into the way she ticks – and the way you tick. Bearing in mind what you have learned about her, decide which of the following categories she fits into, and then read YOUR personality profile, based on hers. You might find your mum fits into more than one category – everyone is unique.

The Perfect Mother ...

The Perfect Mother gets everything right. She's always beautifully turned out, and so young-looking that people take you for sisters. She dresses beautifully and you're never embarrassed to be seen with her. She's careful about her diet, and your diet, filling the house with healthy foods, and providing you and the family with regular, sensible meals, and she sits down and has them with you, eating moderately and sensibly. It's unlikely she's very overweight, and of course she exercises regularly. She tells you to limit your chocolate and keeps an eye on your diet. She has strong views on what you should or shouldn't do. She reads posh magazines to get ideas for new recipes and ways of redecorating the bathroom.

... and you

You wish you could be like your mother and most of the time you reckon you fail. It's lovely to have a mother that your mates envy, but it's a bit tight not to be allowed to pig out on chocolate and crisps occasionally. So you're likely to rebel when she's not around. It's great having a glamorous mum, but it might not be so great when you bring your boyfriend home! You probably feel that your mother worries too much about you, but then she loves you, so she's bound to worry. So if she worries about you, you feel it's your fault, and you wish you could be perfect like her. You might feel a bit dwarfed by your mother, and when you look in the mirror, you're likely to think that you don't measure up to her, but perhaps, if you lost some weight…

The Earth Mother ...

She's indulgent, easy-going and is always in the kitchen. She's possibly overweight, but not necessarily, and her cupboards have cakes, biscuits and other goodies stashed away, for herself and for you. She's the sort of mum who's most likely to cheer you up with chocolate, or to suggest you join her in the kitchen for a snack and a chat. She's cosy and cuddly and your friends envy you because she's so easy to talk to. She does make an effort to look nice, and might wear long skirts and baggy tops, and makes jokes about her weight to show you that she doesn't care. She might be an animal lover, or spend a lot of time helping others. She gives out so much love that sometimes you might even think that she eats so much to replace all the love she's been giving out. She doesn't diet – she says she has no will power. She doesn't bother you about your weight either, and if you complain about being fat, she tells you that you're lovely as you are.

... and you

You probably have your fair share of treats, as that's the way you've been brought up. So you might be a little overweight, especially if the people in your family burn up food slowly. You're close to your mother and love her to bits, but are occasionally embarrassed by her when she comes to your school parents' evening in that tatty old pullover she should have thrown out years ago, and lipstick that doesn't suit her. You think she's the best mum in the world, and you want to be like her when you're a mother, but you don't want to look like her now. It would be nice to be just a little bit slimmer. She thinks you look OK because she loves you, and doesn't see that it's different for you, because you want the boys to fancy you…

The Busy Mother …

Your mum's rushed off her feet. She might work full-time, or be a single parent, or have her own mother to look after, and she simply hasn't got the time to bother about things like her appearance, never wears make-up, and thinks that things like hours spent in the hairdresser are wasted hours. Your mother doesn't have a lot of time to think about food, and there may not be a great deal of food lying about in your house. Your mother doesn't often get the chance to sit down and eat properly as she's so busy, so meals in your house are a bit haphazard. Busy mothers might be overweight because they overeat to give themselves energy, or underweight because they never have time to eat. They're often irritable, complain about not having enough time, and about you not helping more. Watch your busy mum run to the cupboard for her favourite comfort food when the going gets tough.

… and you

You are likely to be quite independent if you have a busy mum, and this could mean that you're quite mature for your age. Also, like your mother, you might feel that it's not very important to care too much about your appearance. A few daughters of very busy mothers might sometimes try dieting or refusing food as a way of demanding attention. Never do that – just tell your mum you want to see more of her. If your mother depends on comfort food to get her through a too-busy day, you might depend on comfort food too. We tend to inherit our mothers' food habits.

The Mixed-up Mother ...

This, I'm afraid, is the largest category. This type of mother has choccy biccies in the cupboard and fat-free butter substitutes in the fridge, diet cola in the pantry and a hoard of Mars bars hidden out of sight. She would love to be half a stone or a stone thinner, tries dieting, makes your life a misery while she's on a diet, until you beg her to eat something – pleease! At other times she comes home from work with cream cakes for everyone because she's pleased with your school report. She reads magazines that tell her what the latest fashions are, and she loves perfume, make-up, and still spends ages getting ready for parties, but can't decide what to wear and asks you for advice. And the most important question is – does she look fat? You assure her she looks lovely but she says she's sure that her stomach is sticking out. She tells you never to diet, but to cut down on your food, and that you are very attractive, but you'd better not put on any more weight. She's got a library of old exercise videos she's stopped using, or an exercise bike in the garage that's gone rusty.

... and you

You've learnt to be sensitive to your mother's mood swings, and enjoy the fact that you're both such good friends. That's why, when she asks you to diet with her, or cut out chocolate together, you're likely to want to do it, and then, when you both can't keep it up any longer, you both pig out. Because your mum is such fun, and so human, you want to be like her, and so you're likely to think of dieting, and likely to look in the mirror and think you're fat, just as she does. To you, all women seem to want to be slimmer, and that seems quite natural. Everyone diets, don't they? You may be hassled by your mother to lose weight, because she still thinks of you as part of her, and you losing weight is almost the same as her getting slimmer. This may seem odd, but mixed-up mums are very peculiar people.

Ten things you're likely to get from your mother

1. Her body shape. Yes, those wide child-bearing hips could be yours, too!

2. Her eating habits. Quick – give me some chocolate somebody, please!

3. Her attitude to her body. If she thinks she's fat, then you'll think you're fat.

4. Her attitude to exercise. If she's a couch potato, she'll write notes to excuse you from swimming if you can't face it.

5. Her attitude to men. If she dresses to impress, she'll teach you how to do that too.

6. Her neuroses. If she worries a lot, you'll probably be a worrier. Mixed-up mums can sometimes bring up mixed-up daughters.

7. Her guilt. If she feels guilty about eating, you'll feel guilty every time you open a packet of crisps.

8. Her diet sheet. Mothers who diet will eventually suggest to their daughters that they try a diet too.

9. Her attitude to fatness. If she thinks it's bad to be fat, you'll grow up believing that too.

10. Love – in the shape of food. When you were a tiny baby (aaahh!) every time you cried, your mother fed you. Many mothers still do.

Help! I've been brainwashed!

Shut up, and eat this biscuit.

No, listen to me. It's very hard if your mother tells you to eat less. You feel you've got no choice.

I understand that. But you do have a choice. One important stage in growing up is learning that you are not your mother. Just because she worries about her weight, it doesn't mean that you have to. Some mothers do tend to see their daughters' bodies as belonging to them – but they don't. On the day you were born, you became a separate person from your mother, and you can now make your own decisions about your appearance and your attitude to your body. Also, don't believe you will grow up entirely like your mother. You won't. You live in a different time from her, and also there's your dad to consider.

Father figures

Oh no – I don't want to look like my dad. A fate worse than death!

With dads, it's more what they say to you. Just as your mum is your female role model, dad is the member of the opposite sex who you know best. Without realizing it, you see him as the spokesman for boys and men everywhere…

My dad's great. Whenever I'm on my way out to a party or somewhere, he wolf-whistles, or makes some joke about making sure I take a bodyguard with me because I'm going to have to fight the boys off. That's never happened yet, but I always feel good when I go out, and even if no boy makes a pass, at least I know my dad loves me!
(Lucy, 15)

This is silly, but whenever I hear my dad go on at my mum about her losing weight, I feel fat. He's never ever told me to go on a diet, and I know he's very proud of me because he's taught me how to play chess and I'm in tournaments with him. I still think he'd like me to lose weight. He must, because Mum's not that fat and he's always telling her to go back to Weight Watchers.
(Jane, 14)

I did go on a diet once, but it only lasted ten days. I exercised a lot too and I lost three pounds. My dad noticed and said I looked gorgeous. I was thrilled. But then it was my birthday, and I had all these chocolates. I put the weight back on. Dad didn't make any comment, but I know he'd be pleased if I lost that weight again. He looked so pleased when I was losing weight, just like he did when I first learned to ride my bike.

(Carly, 13)

Me and my dad watch 'Baywatch' together. He thinks it's dead funny. He laughs at all those fake figures – he calls Pamela Anderson a Barbie doll. I have a laugh too. He says he prefers real women like my mum and he pinches her bum. I think it's embarrassing but she doesn't seem to mind.

(Jeanette, 12)

My dad's never said anything to me about my weight. He's careful not to upset me because I only see him at weekends. But his girlfriend is very slim – she's got a gorgeous figure. My mum's overweight. I know they didn't split up because of that, but it makes you think...

(Leanne, 15)

Which of these dads is a good influence, and which isn't?

Sometimes it's the indirect things dads say that influence you the most. Think about your own dad – has he ever said anything to you about your figure that either upset you, or made you feel good?

Sibling rivalry

Generally dads rarely say cruel things to their daughters. Nor do mums. If you can rely on one person in your family to make a remark as destructive as a thermonuclear explosion, it's going to be your brother or sister. Everybody who has a brother or a sister is going to get called fat at some time in their life. This does not mean you are fat. I repeat, THIS DOES NOT MEAN YOU ARE FAT. Check out the list below to find out the most common reason why your brother or sister calls you fat…

1. Your brother loves teasing you. It makes him feel powerful when he can rile you and see you lose your cool. Try not reacting next time he calls you fatso. Just agree with him happily. He won't have a clue what to do next.

2. Your sister wants to borrow your slinky black dress. She knows if she mentions that your stomach sticks out when you wear it, you'll wear something else for the party you're both going to. Underhand, isn't she?

3. Your brother is very fond of you. Like most

blokes, it's hard for him to say that. So he does the opposite. He pretends he doesn't love you by calling you names. 'Fat' is as good as any other. He's very surprised when you don't like it, because he thought you knew he didn't mean it. These are the sort of brothers who regularly fail intelligence tests.

4. Your sister is furious with you because you've grabbed the best armchair for watching *Home and Away*/have taken the last chocolate digestive/won't do her maths homework for her/won't let her listen to your tape of the latest East 17 single. (Delete as applicable.) So she calls you fat. It's guaranteed to hurt. Revenge is sweet!

5. All your brother's mates go on about how gorgeous Pamela Anderson is, and your stupid brother actually believes all girls are meant to look like that. Boy, is he going to be disappointed! So he informs you that you're fat. Treat this with the contempt it deserves.

6. Your sister tells you you're fat because she's on a diet. OK, so this is not logical, but then, the first thing dieters lose is their logic, not those extra pounds. Your sister's so hungry most of the time that she gets irritable and takes it out on little ol' you, who's happily sitting down with a delicious chicken and mushroom pie.

Now come on, do you *really* believe everything your brothers and sisters tell you? Of course you don't. So don't react too strongly if they call you fat. They can't help it, poor things.

So who should you listen to, when it comes to weight? If your family's advice is not always well-judged, what about society itself? Should you pay close attention to the magazines you read or the actresses and models you admire?

Chapter 4

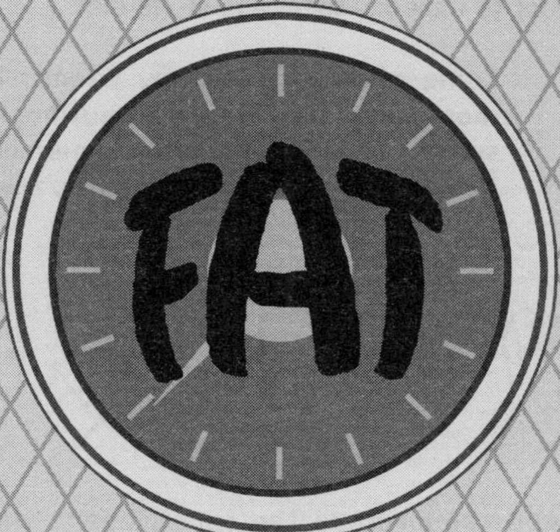

Role models and supermodels

The supermodel debate

Girls who don't need to lose weight are pressured into dieting because of the supermodels. All of them – Cindy Crawford, Claudia Schiffer, Naomi Campbell, Kate Moss – are pencil thin. We want to look like them and so we diet.

Come off it. Me and my friends have more sense than to pin all our hopes of success on looking like the supermodels. I don't want to be a clothes horse, anyway.

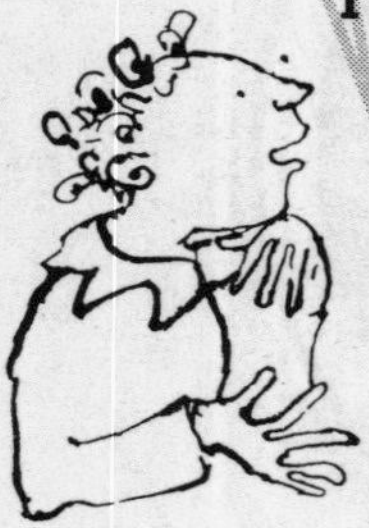

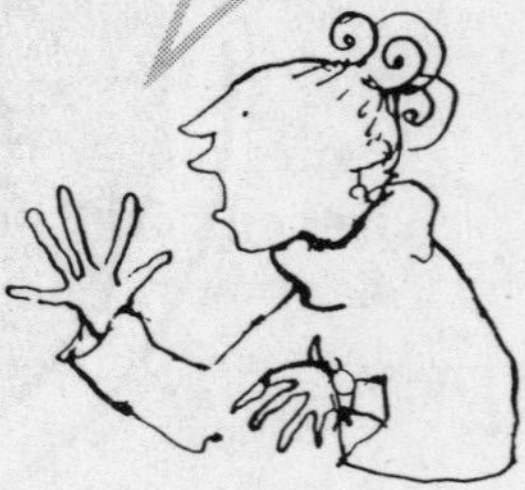

But you can't escape the supermodels. They're everywhere you go, and the pictures of them get under our skin. I don't believe any girl who says she wouldn't exchange her body with Naomi Campbell.

Yeah – I'd like to win the lottery too but I know I'm not going to. I also know I'm never going to look like Naomi Campbell so I don't let it bother me.

Everybody looks up to the supermodels. They have such a brilliant time – the magazines I read are full of stories about the parties they go to and their boyfriends and husbands. And they're rich.

They're freaks of nature. Nobody, but nobody, has a body like Kate Moss naturally. I'd love to shove a decent size meal down her.

But Kate Moss doesn't diet. It's not her fault for being slim and beautiful. Just like it's not a clever person's fault for being top in maths. I really like Kate Moss and I hate it when people blame her for something she can't help.

So because you like her, you want to look like her? I like my boyfriend, but I don't want to look like him!

The models are there to show us what people consider to be beautiful. It's like a guideline for us.

I prefer to make up my own mind about how I should look, thank you very much.

Yes. But what if you think you look good and nobody else does? Then all your mates will laugh at you.

So at least I bring happiness into other people's lives!

What do *you* think? Are the supermodels to blame for the rising numbers of girls suffering from eating disorders? Are they to blame every time you look in the mirror and throw your hands up in despair at what you see?

Here's Sandi Dalton, a 14-year-old model working in Manchester, on her first-hand experience of the modelling industry.

I've always wanted to be a model, and so one day I went into a model agency on spec, to get them to assess my potential. Of the forty of us that went in for an assessment session, only three of us were told we had what it takes, and I was one of them. I was thrilled to bits, although my mum was worried because I'm still at school. The agency put me on a course, where I learnt how to walk down a catwalk, photographics, make-up and confidence building. Then we had a sort of graduation ceremony with judges and everything. After that you're put on the agency's books, and you get offered real modelling assignments. I've been given the chance to work in New York and to audition for a soap opera.

When I first started the course, I was measured. I'm 5′ 8″, and my vital statistics were 34-24-38. I was told I had to lose inches off my hips. I was given exercises to do every day. I lost two inches off my hips, but really that isn't enough. With my statistics, I wouldn't get work in Japan – there they want really flat-chested, petite, small-hipped models. I wasn't given a diet as such, just these exercises.

I'm one of the youngest models at the agency. I don't smoke, but most of the older ones do. I know it's because they worry about their weight, and they need to keep slim. I guess there are quite a few anorexics, although I don't know for sure. I can honestly say that there are some models I work with who I never see eat! In the agency we know that at the moment gaunt is 'in' and all the older models – some of them have children – have to work really hard to keep unnaturally thin. I'm lucky I'm at school because it gives me a sense of proportion – I know it's important to get good exam results too.

I think it's small-minded of girls to model themselves on people like Kate Moss. You're either like her or you're not like her. Different people have different bone structures. I have to say that I think the really ultra-thin models like Jodie Kidd look awful – I've never spoken to anyone who likes the way she looks, or met any boy who fancies her. The lads are really rude about Jodie Kidd.

Modelling is a job just like any other. To be a model, you've got to be reasonably slim, just like you've got to have a degree to be a doctor. I think it's wrong to blame models for making girls obsessive about their weight. The way I see it, when a girl discovers that a boy she fancies doesn't fancy her, she can't accept it, so she focuses on her weight. That's not my fault.

Models - the vital statistics

1. Victorian Vamps!

Back in the bad old Victorian days (when girls weren't allowed to even speak to a boy who wasn't her brother until she had her parents' permission) there were still role models for females. There were magazines – one was even edited by Charles Dickens – that wrote about women's lives, and had drawings of the ideal woman of that time. She had a decent-sized bust, a teeny weeny waist, and wore crinoline dresses over whalebone frames, so she could afford to have quite big hips. In Victorian times a tiny waist was to die for – literally. Women and girls squeezed themselves into bone corsets and got their maids to tie them in to them as tightly as they could. No wonder Victorian women were prone to having fainting fits – the poor loves could hardly breathe. Victorian men liked tiny waists and big hips because a) it meant the woman they fancied wasn't pregnant by any other man and b) if she had big hips, she'd probably be good at having babies – and Victorian menfolk were keen on big families. Queen Victoria had nine children.

2. Edwardians? – Bum-tastic!

After 1900, the fashions changed. Women rushed out to their nearest emporiums and bought the bustle, which was –

wait for it – an artificial bum they stuck on their behind, so that when they walked along the street, their behinds could be admired from behind. The bigger the bum, the better.

3. Flat-chested Flappers

In the 1920s, women with tiny waists and large hips suddenly found themselves out of fashion. After the First World War, when women had taken over men's jobs as the men were away fighting, women felt they'd had enough just being child-bearers and wanted to have fun, fun, fun – like the men! Fashions changed. Dresses got shorter, hair was bobbed, and thin was in. Flapper girls – so called after their hairstyles – had no boobs to speak of, and their figures went straight up and down like boys' figures. They smoked using cigarette holders and wore make-up – thoroughly modern young misses. Things that we call 'gross' they called 'utterly sick-making' and where we'd say 'cool' now, they said 'too, too sweet!'.

4. Food for Snappers

Over in the US of A at the same time, photography was taking off in a big way. Fashion houses wanted photographers to take pictures of their latest designs on beautiful women, which would naturally make their clothes look more beautiful still. Enter the fashion model! Like the Victorian Miss, she tended to have boobs, a tiny waist and hips that came out. Her legs weren't too important then, as skirts tended to cover them. The first models walked the streets of Manhattan with their little hat boxes containing all their make-up, going where their agencies sent them, in pursuit of dollars earned posing for the camera. The most successful models were highly sought after, but weren't as famous as…

5. Screen Queens

In the 1930s, 40s and 50s women all over the West wanted to look like the film stars that paraded on their cinema screens. To be cool like Lauren Bacall! To have eyes like Bette Davis! To have legs like Betty Grable! Boobs like Jayne Mansfield! And the greatest Screen Goddess of them all was Marilyn Monroe. She had shapely – and not small – breasts, a waist that went in, but came straight out again swelling into curvaceous hips, and fleshy, shapely legs. Marilyn Monroe wore the American dress size 12 (British size 16), and was not thin. Definitely not thin. Men lusted after her, and women envied her, because she was shapely. In the fifties, girls and women dyed their hair blonde to look like her, padded their bras, and slicked on the lippy. And the men of Britain stood and drooled.

6. Twiggy and the twiglets

Something happened in the 1960s. Swinging London was where it was at, and a young fashion photographer discovered a new model – not a glamorous film star but a chirpy little Cockney: Twiggy. Where Marilyn Monroe went out and in and out, Twiggy just went down in one straight line – all the better to model the new shift dresses and tiny mini-skirts that were all the rage at that time. Twiglets like Twiggy parted their hair in the middle, grew it dead straight – ironing it on their mum's ironing board if it was frizzy – wore boob tubes to hide their boobs – and their dads shouted at them for wearing skirts so short that every time they bent down folk could see their behinds.

Was it just a spooky coincidence that Weight Watchers, the first of the slimming clubs, came to Britain at this time?

7. Supermodels reign supreme

Perhaps television had something to do with it, but after the 1960s, film stars didn't have quite so much influence with us. It was models who seemed to be having all the fun, who were at all the trendy parties, who married all the rock stars, and who decorated the pages of all the magazines. Girls everywhere dreamed of being models, despite the hard work involved, and the poor rate of pay at the lower end of the market. Increasingly fewer and fewer women were being paid more and more and more, and getting all the top assignments – the supermodels. Hello – Cindy Crawford, Elle McPherson, Christy Turlington, Claudia Schiffer, Naomi Campbell and Kate Moss. And since 1967, statistics show that models' vital statistics are getting smaller – thin is in.

Why is thin in?

- Today's outrageous fashions hang better on thinner models.
- Television cameras make a woman look about ten pounds fatter, so it helps if a model is underweight.
- Men like the vulnerable little girl look, and little girls don't have a woman's shape.
- The Shock Factor. If a fashion company gets an ultra-thin-look!-you-can-see-her-bones!-yeuch!-isn't-she-revolting? model for their new collection, all the papers will splash pictures over their front pages, and the fashion company's new styles get nationwide coverage.
- It's a conspiracy. One day the supermodels are going to vanish entirely!

Round the world survey ... Round the world survey ... Round the world survey ... Round the world survey ... Round the world

- 90 per cent of all cultures consider fat hips and thighs to be attractive in women.
- Thinness in women is most common in Japan, China, England and France.
- In many countries fatness in women is seen as desirable, and some brides are fattened up for their weddings.
- Jamaican men prefer women with 'shape' to thin women.

So who's beautiful? The answer depends where and when you're living! All well and good – except most of us can't emigrate to that island paradise where the women everyone fancies are size 16 at least. Most of us are stuck here in the West in the 1990s. And the pressure is on us to look good. Except there's a mystery here. No one ever tells the under-18s to lose weight. There are no television programmes for fourteen-year-olds who want to diet. Teen magazines never advise all their readers to lose weight. The supermodels just do their jobs – they don't wear placards saying *Girls – look like me!* So how come we all feel we should all be slimmer?

In a random survey conducted on 28 15 to 16-year-old girls of average weight, 22 out of 28 said they wanted to be slimmer.

So where does this pressure come from?

Elementary, my dear Watson! Allow me to explain.

Clue number one: In our society, men are seen as the strong, protective sex, and women as the soft, gentle, nurturing sex. In most pictures of men and women in the West, men are shown as bigger than women. Look at old family portraits, and you will often see women sitting down and men standing up. Big women were seen to pose a threat to the social order.

But, Holmes, I don't see...

Clue number two: Whenever we see a picture of an ideal woman, she is not too big – she's slim, in fact. It doesn't matter if she's too slim – the important thing is that she's not too big.

Yes, but...

Clue number three: So! If you are trying to sell a product – say, for example, a shampoo, and you wish to show a woman using it, you choose an ideal woman – one that will make you think, if I buy and use this shampoo, I will look like this ideal woman. Inevitably, this ideal woman will be slim.

So slim women are used to sell things...

Clue number four: Look around you. There are television, cinemas, magazines, newspapers, advertising hoardings, advertising leaflets, posters – and on all of them slim women are selling things. So a typical girl, in a single day, might very well see more ideal women on television, in magazines, in the cinema than she might see in real life, thus leading to a confusion between the ideal and the real.

Slow down, will you? I'm confused now.

I repeat – we are bombarded with images of slim women everywhere, so we begin to believe that this is normal. We forget that all around us in the real world are girls of all different shapes and sizes. We believe that television and magazines tell us the truth. But they do not.

Clue number five: Everybody wants to be normal. But we no longer compare ourselves to normal people, only to the images of ideal women we see. So naturally we feel we should be slimmer, more beautiful, have silkier hair…

I see! So the real villains are the industries that sell us things using glamorous models. They make us feel inadequate.

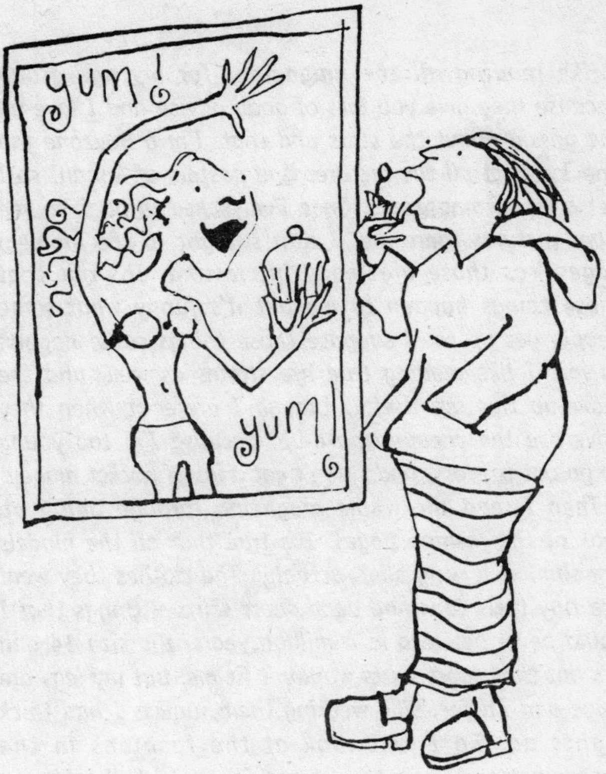

Congratulations, my dear Watson. At last you have it. Did you know that in Scandinavia the use of real people in advertisements is illegal?

And yet … if our manufacturers started advertising their products using normal-looking models, would people still buy them? If 50-year-old Mrs Jones down your road was on the box telling you how the latest perfume *Mysteria* made her smell like a bed of roses, would you buy it? If the latest teen fashions were modelled by a girl who was lacking in the looks department, would you want to buy that skirt she was wearing? Honestly, now!

'I like reading all the magazines for my age group because they give you lots of good advice and I love all the gossip about the stars and that. I'm a Boyzone fan and I collect all the pictures and posters of Ronan, so I get a lot of magazines. Once I've flicked through to see what pictures there are, I turn straight to the problem pages 'cos those are really interesting. It's not that those things happen to me but it's funny what some people get up to. I suppose those things could happen to me. I like reading true life stories as well, and the make-up tips are useful, though I prefer it when they advertise the cheaper make-up, because I'm too young to go out to work, and I don't get a lot of pocket money.

Then I read the whole magazine through and I do look at the fashion pages. It's true that all the models are slim, well, very slim, actually. The clothes they wear are tiny little tops and dead short skirts – things that I could never get into in a million years. I'm size 14 and it's not that short skirts wouldn't fit me, but my legs are huge and I'd feel silly wearing them, unless I had thick tights on. So I just look at the fashions in the magazines and know they're not for me. I feel a bit out of it – it's like there's all those other readers who can wear those fashions, and then there's me.

But I tell you what gets me. You read the problem pages and there are letters sometimes from girls saying that they're worried that they're fat, and the answer always tells them not to worry because it's personality that counts, and it's the person inside that matters, and all that kind of thing, and you turn over the page, and there are all thin models wearing the latest fashions, or posing in the photo-story pictures. It's like a kind of double message.

What's even worse is when they have these special spreads with fat models, like they're freaks that can only be allowed on special pages. Why can't they have fatter models alongside the ordinary ones, and not separate the two? And why can't the fashion designers come up with some fashions for bigger girls? Most of the things in my magazines suit my little sister more than me. ***(Claire, 13)***

Chapter 5

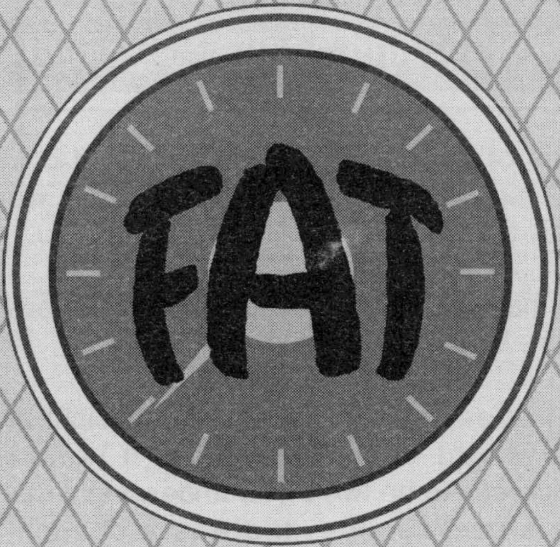

What you're eating and what's eating you

But it's unhealthy to be fat, isn't it? That's why it's important to do something about it. My mum says it's bad for me to be overweight and I've got to eat healthily. Health is the most important thing.

Weight and health – the facts

- Many of the doctors' warnings about being fat causing poor health applies to older women, rarely to teenagers.
- You have to be a good three stone overweight before it seriously affects your health.
- It's just as unhealthy to be underweight as it is overweight – for a teenager, it is *far more dangerous* to be two stone underweight than two stone overweight – there is a chance your periods won't function properly.
- Obesity is not an illness – caused, for example, by viruses or bacteria – it's a condition.
- To tell if your excess weight is affecting you, ask yourself if you are out of breath when walking upstairs, whether exercise is difficult, and whether you have pain in your joints. If you can answer 'yes' to two of those questions, your weight may be causing you a health problem.

- Doctors sometimes tell you to lose weight not because you are ill, but because your weight is above average according to their weight tables. They wouldn't suggest you chop eight centimetres off if you were too tall. Remember, doctors aren't gods; they're only human beings.

- A great deal of excess weight might make it difficult for a surgeon to operate on you, but not impossible.

- Your fertility (ability to have a baby) is much more likely to be damaged by excess dieting than excess weight.

- The condition called osteoporosis ('brittle bones') is more likely to be caused by malnutrition than by eating too much.

- A high cholesterol level (the gooey stuff that can clog up your arteries in later life) isn't related to how fat you are.

- No scientist has ever been able to prove a direct link between fat and illness. Being slightly fat doesn't make you ill.

- There are certain health conditions that improve if you aren't carrying extra weight. These are high blood pressure, arthritis, heart disease and late onset diabetes. If you are very healthy, but overweight, then you are still very healthy.

- Far, far more important than what weight you are, is what you eat, and how much exercise you take. Throw away those scales and get yourself a mountain bike!
- Fat produces oestrogens, which protect against heart disease and brittle bones.

I never eat breakfast. The thought of it makes me sick and I haven't got the time. Actually, I don't eat much at school. But in the evenings I keep picking.
(Anna, 14)

I'm a vegetarian and I know it's important to eat a balanced diet. My mum gets me all those ready prepared meals from the supermarket. I know they're not cheap but at least she knows I'm eating properly.
(Emma, 15)

All right – I admit it. I'm addicted to chocolate. When I go past the choccy machine at school it's like it's a big magnet, and it's pulling me, pulling me. In goes the money my dad gave me for lunch. I just can't resist. Help!
(Joanna, 14)

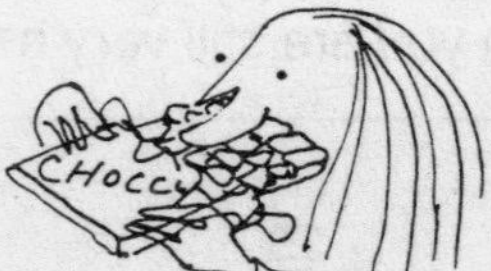

I don't have a set pattern of eating. Like, if I'm going to a party or out with my mates, I never feel like having much, especially if I'm going to be meeting boys. But if I'm staying in all day or I'm bored, then I'll eat loads – biscuits, sandwiches, anything.
(Debbie, 15)

I won't eat vegetables. Well, no, that's not absolutely true. I do eat peas and sweetcorn. But that's all. My mum and dad nag me about it but broccoli – yeauch! I couldn't eat it to save my life. Well, maybe to save my life – but I'll be sick after...
(Jan, 13)

I don't like eating in other people's houses. I like my mum's cooking but I really have to force myself to eat if I'm staying at a friend's. Even at home, I just like plain food. I've never had a curry ever. I don't want to try one.
(Sam, 12)

My mum makes sure I eat a healthy diet. I have muesli in the morning and she gives me lots of fruit in my lunch box, and just one chocolate biscuit. I have a proper meal at home with meat and two veg, and sometimes we have a dessert. I have a hot drink before bed. I'm only allowed chocolate on chocolate days, which are Friday and Sunday.
(Katharine, 13)

I take fruit to have with my lunch but I swap it with my friend's Snickers.
(Nasreen, 12)

My mum gives me a packed lunch but I throw it away. I don't want to get fat.
(Lissa, 15)

So what's normal? What do teenage girls eat in a typical day? Here are some real menus from three typical 15-year-old girls – none of them significantly overweight.

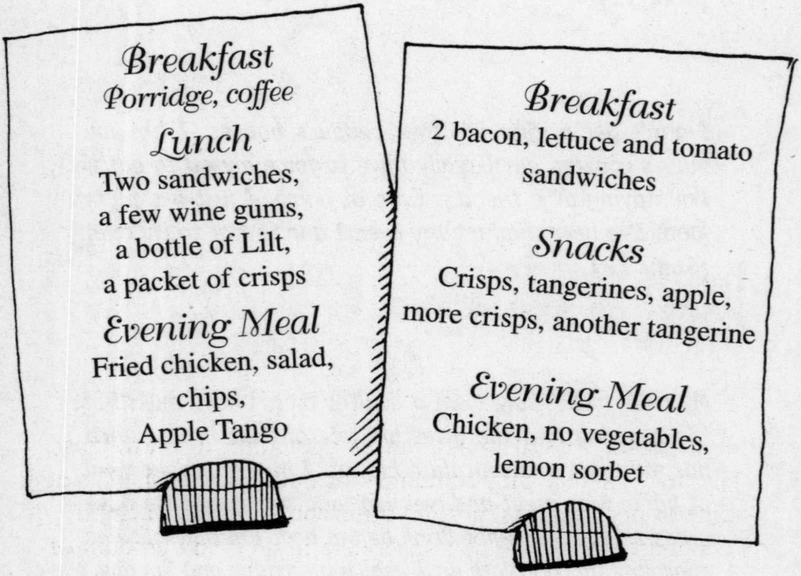

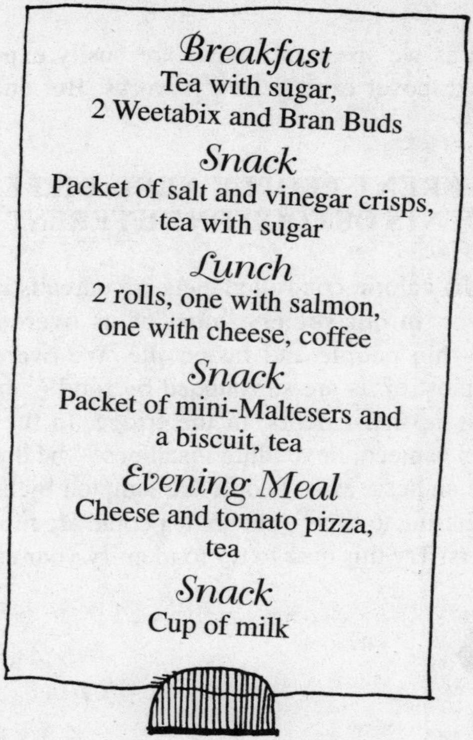

> Girls need 15-18 per cent of their body weight to consist of fat if they are to grow breasts and become fertile.

Most people's food intake varies depending on how busy they are, whether they're hungry or not, whether they're at home or not, and on a million different emotional factors. People are not cars. They don't take in a certain amount of fuel at fixed times, run out, grind to a standstill, and then need filling up. Our appetite is a delicate, irregular thing, and even as we speak, scientists are busily experimenting trying to discover exactly how it works. But one thing we do know –

DIFFERENT PEOPLE NEED DIFFERENT AMOUNTS OF FOOD ON DIFFERENT DAYS.

This is why calorie-controlled diets are unrealistic.

However, in our society, most of us overeat to some degree – thin people and fat people. We overeat simply because most of us are surrounded by food – in shops, on television advertisements, in the fridge, in the pantry, in the school canteen, in vending machines – the opportunities to eat are endless. Most people are tempted by high-calorie food from time to time – but some people are more tempted than others. Try this quiz to try to identify your eating type.

Quiz

1. You're out with your mates and pass a chippy. You can smell the chips and you…

a) feel slightly sick. All that fat!

b) think it might be nice to get some but you'd prefer to spend your hard-earned dosh on something else.

c) go in on impulse. Chips are scrummy-yummy. You offer to treat your friends.

2. You're staying in, waiting for *him* to ring. The phone remains silent all evening. By 10 pm…

a) you have a good weep and vow to give up boys for ever.

b) you have a good weep, vow to give up boys for ever,

and have three choccy biccies and a hot cocoa.

c) you open the pantry, get out an unopened packet of biscuits, consume them, take handfuls of *Coco-Pops* and consume them, see if there are any crisps left, and eat what you can find. Feel sick, hate yourself, and go to bed.

3. You're revising for your History exam. It's not hard but it's boring. So you…

a) have a break, listen to the radio, then force yourself to start again.

b) go and look in the fridge, find yesterday's apple pie, cut yourself a slice, and take it back to your room with a cup of tea.

c) pop down to the corner shop, buy loads of Jelly Babies, an Uncle Tom's Mint Ball, a bar of chocolate and get stuck in.

4. Your friends are coming round to watch a video. You prepare by…

a) getting the video from the shop.

b) asking your mum if you can pop some oven chips in the oven later on.

c) getting the video from the shop, and buying lots of popcorn and other goodies to share with your mates, secretly hoping they're not that hungry. You don't really enjoy a film unless you can eat while you watch it.

5. Everyone's out and there's nothing to do. You are so *bored* you could *SCREEEAM!* So you…

a) screeeam!

b) wonder what there is to eat in the house.

c) go and find out what there is to eat in the house, make a huge pile of food, and take it back to your room.

6. You're out at the shops with your mum, but you haven't been able to find anything you like. As a consolation you buy…

a) a magazine to read.
b) a *Time Out* bar.
c) as much choccy as your mum will allow you.

7. It's your birthday! Happy birthday! Your best mate buys you a box of chocolates. You…

a) put them away for later. In a few days you open it and have just one.
b) thank her warmly, open it, offer her some, and the two of you devour the lot, with a bit of help from mum and dad and little sister.
c) put it away for later. Then when no one is around, you scoff the lot.

8. As far as dessert is concerned…

a) you have it if there's any going.
b) you always like to have some and prefer pudding, but will happily eat fruit or yoghurt.
c) you always insist on it and have seconds if you can.

9. When you wake up in the morning, you…

a) think about what's happening that day.
b) think about what's happening that day and wonder what there is for breakfast.
c) feel dreadful about what you ate last night, and think about what you will/won't eat today.

10. You eat sweets…

a) rarely or never.
b) in the car when you're bored, but not that often.
c) all the time.

Results

Mostly a)s.

You eat to live. Food plays a very small part in your life, and you spend very little time thinking about it, unless you're hungry. It's unlikely you'll ever have a problem with food or weight, unless you deliberately stop yourself from eating.

Mostly b)s.

You love to eat. And what's wrong with that? Most healthy people with a keen appetite enjoy eating, and eat to celebrate, or cheer themselves up. In moderation, comfort eating or boredom eating won't do you much harm. It's absolutely normal.

Mostly c)s.

You live to eat. It's possible that you do eat too much. Although the idea of a binge is appealing and it sometimes feels as if it might be the answer to your problems, binges always backfire. They leave you feeling disgusted with yourself and out of control. If you really feel overeating is a problem, have a look at the chapter on eating disorders.

So what should you eat? As you can see, there's no simple answer. Everyone is different. A good guideline, however, is the food triangle.

		Examples
Don't have too many of these	FATS OILS ADDED SUGAR	Crisps, chocolate, sweets, greasy take-aways
Eat moderate but regular amounts of these	FISH, POULTRY, MEAT, EGGS, MILK, BEANS, CHEESE, NUTS	Yogurts, roast chicken, fish fingers, grilled beefburger, baked beans
Have plenty of these	FRUIT, VEGETABLES	Apples, bananas, oranges, cabbage, carrots, cauliflower
Eat your fill!	BREAD, PASTA, RICE POTATOES, CEREALS	Spaghetti, noodles, bran flakes, weetabix, porridge

If you generally keep to these proportions in your daily diet, you won't go far wrong. Vegetarians need to know just a little bit more about nutrition than the rest of us, as they have to check they're getting enough first class protein. It can be healthy to be a veggie, but they're not immune from putting on weight – veggies eat chocolate too!

Chapter 6

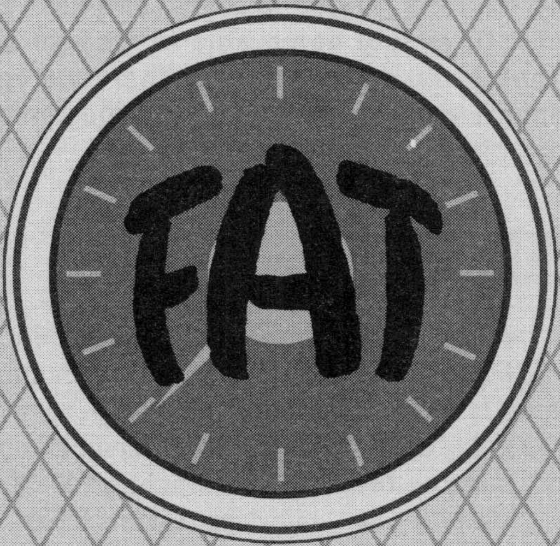

Tempted to diet? Don't try it!

'To diet, or not to diet, that is the question. Whether 'tis nobler in the mind…'

Oh, shut up! It's not funny. I've read everything so far and I'm still not happy with the way I look. The plain fact is I'm overweight. I know I'd look better if I was slimmer. I want to go on a diet. I dream of being really slim, of boys giving me long, lingering looks, and girls being jealous. Or simply being able to fit into a size 10. That would do for starters. That, and having a stomach that doesn't stick out. You can't talk me out of it – I'm going on a diet…

What is a diet?

'Diet' is one of the most misused words in the English language. 'Diet' simply means a food plan, nothing more and nothing less. But what most people mean when they say they're going on a diet is that they're going to cut down their food intake in order to lose weight. Probably they're going to stick to a plan, and deprive themselves of high-calorie food.

> In 1991, we Britons spent £90 million on frozen 'slimmer's' meals.

These days, we hear a lot about healthy eating. What's that? It's respecting your body by not shovelling it full of junk food. Everybody, whether they're fat, thin or in between, should eat healthily – see the food triangle in the previous chapter.

So what's the difference between healthy eating and dieting? Some diet commercials try to kid you that their diet is the same as healthy eating. Not in my book they're not.

My definitions:

DIETING IS WHEN YOU EAT LESS THAN YOU NEED IN ORDER TO LOSE WEIGHT.

HEALTHY EATING IS WHEN YOU SATISFY YOUR HUNGER BY EATING NUTRITIOUS, WELL BALANCED FOOD.

You can't do both at once. If you are dieting you are eating less than you need, and therefore you can't be getting all your nutritional requirements. Don't let dieting organizations kid you – wise up! So do you still want to go on a diet?

I do. I told you – I want to lose weight.

OK – it's a free country.

13 weird and wonderful ways to lose weight from the past and present

1. **Banting** – not eating starchy food, a method invented by a London undertaker (spooky or what?).

2. **Every Woman's Flesh Reducer** – taking a bath with citric acid, Epsom salts, camphor, soda and alum (let's hope your boyfriend doesn't have a sense of smell).

3. **Absorbit Reducing Paste** – you spread this all over your body. It contains oxbile, beeswax and lard.

4. **Fatoff** – a paste which was 10 per cent soap and 90 per cent water to rub into those fleshy regions.

5. **Enemas** – this time a soapy solution is injected into your back passage – bet you can guess the result!

6. **Electric Shocks** – I kid you not.

7. **Body Wraps** – you wrap yourself in silver foil and wait till you get slimmer. You lose lots of fluid, but one glass of water and the weight's back on again.

8. **DNTP** – a substance that raised the body's metabolic rate (burns your calories faster).

Trouble was, it also led to blindness, deafness and death. A rather drastic way to lose weight.

9. **Bai Lin Tea** – drink this herbal tea, promised the manufacturers, and the weight will just drop off. Needless to say, it didn't work.

10. **The Mayo Diet** – you only eat tomato juice and hard boiled eggs – with the shells off, of course. Too many calories in those.

11. **AYDS** – you chewed these vile-tasting spongy cubes before each meal, and they were supposed to reduce your appetite. Desperate slimmers ate them like sweets and – wait for it – got fatter.

12. **The Tapeworm Diet** – as tried by the opera singer Maria Callas. Squeamish readers – stop here. Callas swallowed a tablet containing an embryonic tapeworm which grew inside her and ate all her food. Yes, a fully-grown tapeworm lived in her stomach.

13. **The Amphetamine Diet** – many women were given, and are still being given, amphetamines to lose weight. These drugs are known in the drug world as speed – you might lose your appetite but you might also shake uncontrollably, feel neurotic and be unable to sleep.

OK, OK, I'm not that desperate. But I know there are lots of easier and pleasanter ways to diet because there are advertisements everywhere, and diet books, and slimming clubs, and...

Slimming clubs

I'm not so much fat, as small. I had this idea that if I dieted I'd look taller. Since my mum dieted all the time, she was quite happy for me to diet with her.

When she thought about joining Weight Watchers she asked me to go with her as she didn't like the thought of going on her own. I was twelve, or maybe thirteen then. When I asked if I could join they asked me what my reasons were, so I explained about my mum. They asked me if I had anorexia or bulimia and I said no. They didn't ask me to see my doctor or anything. Then they gave me a booklet about what I should eat. It was quite complicated and I sat there reading it for ages. Because of my age they didn't give me a target weight although my mum got one. I was given a food diary, though, in which I had to write down everything I ate.

I sort of stuck to it, and they weighed me once or twice a month. But the meetings were silly, they didn't tell you anything you didn't already know. We both stopped going after a time, although we do try to keep to the guidelines they gave us. I didn't lose any weight.
(Trish, 14)

Weight Watchers, Slimming World, The Rosemary Conley Diet and Fitness Centres, are examples of slimming clubs. You go once a week for advice about food intake, to get weighed, and be encouraged to stay with the diet. You have to pay a sum of money every week, even paying if you skip a meeting. Current weekly fees are around £4–£5. The diets they give you are complicated, and do involve you eating fewer calories than you need in order to lose weight. The thing to remember about slimming clubs is that they are profit-making companies: you want to lose pounds; they want to gain pounds – your pounds – pounds sterling, that is. That's their main reason for existing. If they can make dieting addictive, they will do. All the more money for them.

> In 1992 Weight Watchers' 3,000 or so branches made a PROFIT of £20 million pounds. They certainly put on more than they lost!

Meal replacements

I wanted to try Slimfast because it looked so easy. You just have these drinks and don't bother about anything else. Then in the evening you can have a proper meal. My mum said I could give it a try as long as I didn't get too hungry. We got the chocolate flavour ones as they looked delicious.

The first morning it was fun, having a milk shake for breakfast. By lunchtime I was starving, and when I was making up the shake in the school canteen everyone was staring. I was glad I was on a diet. It didn't fill me up. I was still hungry all through double maths. I felt a bit weepy when I got home but Mum said she'd poached some salmon for me. I had that and felt better.

All the next day I was weak from hunger. I had a headache at school but also a funny sickly feeling that meant I wasn't that hungry. That was good. On the third day I was hungry again and I felt so jealous of all my friends having sandwiches for lunch – really jealous. In the end I wanted food more than I wanted to be slim. On the way back from school I went in the newsagent and bought a packet of crisps. I've never enjoyed a packet of crisps more in my life. I went home and told my mum. She was a bit angry because she'd bought all the Slimfast, but she said it was just as well because she thought I was beginning to look peaky. ***(Sara, 15)***

Slimfast is an example of a meal substitute. There are lots of these now in supermarkets and chemist shops. They might be powders to put in liquid, or even chocolate biscuits. They are meant to replace a whole meal, and they're supposed to contain all the vitamins and minerals you need. In fact, they are full of artificial chemicals. Anyone who's tried them will tell you they are not as filling as a real meal, and may make you feel slightly ill. They are also pricey – surely the Slimfast manufacturers aren't also after a quick buck?

> A typical low-calorie meal replacement has as many calories as a Mars bar.
> (I know which one I'd prefer!)

Calorie counting

I bought this book with my birthday money which tells you exactly how many calories there are in everything you eat. I decided to stick to 1,200 calories a day. It seemed like a lot. But it wasn't – by the evening I'd eaten most of them and I was still hungry. That wasn't the worst part. I didn't mind being hungry, but it was all the adding up of the calories. It was, like, 45 for an apple, and 135 for bread and butter, 15 for a mint and so on, and I'm in the bottom set for maths. All these figures going around my head. I got fed up with it in the end. ***(Rochelle, 15)***

A calorie is just a unit of energy – the more calories that are in your food, the more energy you are consuming. Energy you don't use turns into fat. So in calorie-controlled diets you take in less energy than you need – hardly a recipe to make you feel good. Also, you need to take a calculator with you everywhere!

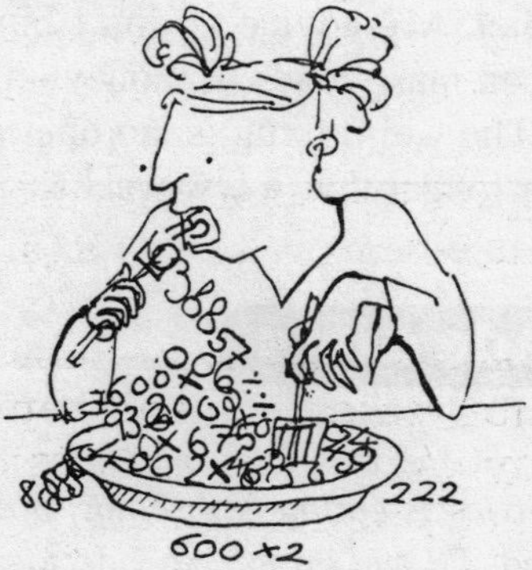

Diet books

My mum had a book called 'The F-Plan', I think it was. She said we would have the meals in that, because they were all high in fibre and low in calories. They were revolting! All that fibre gives you wind, and there was one evening when she'd made a bean stew type thing, and my boyfriend called round after. I was sitting with my legs crossed all the time!

I didn't stick to it. I refused to eat the meals and anyway, at school I had normal school dinners. But my mum kept at it and wouldn't even go out with my dad for a meal on her birthday. She lost about a stone. That was last year. She's put it back on again now.

(Carly, 15)

Every few months, a new diet book hits the bookshops. These books contain success stories of people who have tried these diets, reasons why they are good for you, and lists of what you should eat every day, together with recipes. Mums like them because they take the thought out of planning a diet. My advice is don't buy a diet book – write one. You can make loads of money – they sell like hot cakes. (Sorry!) The weird thing is, no one ever sticks to the diets in them for longer than a few weeks.

Home-made diets

I just thought I was eating bad things, and if I went on as I was doing, I'd end up fat. So I decided to cut down my crisps to one packet a week, and eat lots of apples. I also made myself eat breakfast – I like Rice Krispies. Oh yes, and I cut out milk. I drank water instead.

At first I was excited because I thought I'd lose loads of weight. I got more conscious of food, and every time I saw someone else eating chocolate, which I wouldn't allow myself, I got jealous. Because it was my cousin's party in a week, I wanted to be slim for that, and I was thinking about not eating, and getting slim, all the time. I didn't starve myself, but eventually I just went back to eating the old way. I don't know if it's because I haven't got any will power. I'd still like to be slim and I might diet again. But I like food. It's hard, isn't it? ***(Jane, 13)***

Just cutting back what you're eating is something nearly all of us have tried. We all know that we shouldn't eat too many crisps, chocolate and thick peanut butter sandwiches. Yet whenever you try to deprive yourself of something you want, it has a funny effect on your mind. You keep thinking about what you can't have, so you end up wanting it more than you did before. No, you're not mad. This happens to everyone.

Slimming meals

My dad and I went on this diet when he bought those Lean Cuisine meals from the supermarket and we had one of those each in the evening. I liked them. They were nice. I got hungry later on, and when my dad was upstairs working, I used to nick some biscuits. In the end he stopped getting them, because he said they were too expensive. It was a shame, as I liked the pasta ones. ***(Leanne, 14)***

Lean Cuisine and Heinz/Weight Watchers make whole meals for dieters, which are calorie counted. Many busy parents buy them. But did you know that they are just as high in fat as similar meals that don't claim to be diet meals? When you're in the supermarket, beware. Foods that are labelled 'reduced fat' or even 'low in fat' may not be. Who says what is low and what is high? There's no law about this.

A Food Commission survey discovered that a supermarket's Healthy Eating burgers were nearly a third as expensive as their normal burgers.

Ways to lose weight that no one should ever try

- ✖ **Very Low Calorie Diets** (for example, the Cambridge Diet). These are not for teenagers and can cause malnutrition.

- **Skipping meals.** You need food. Your body is not designed to run without it.

- **Smoking.** Some people actually start smoking because they think they will lose weight. Do you really want to be a thin corpse? Lung cancer is also a jolly good way to lose weight, and that's one proven result of smoking.

- **Taking laxatives** (pills that send you running to the loo). This way you lose vital nutrients and you don't lose weight because your body has already absorbed the food you've taken in.

- **Liposuction.** This is an operation, carried out under general anaesthetic, when your fat is painfully sucked out of your body down a long tube. I wonder where they put it all afterwards? The operation leaves you swollen, bruised and uncomfortable. And it doesn't stop you putting on weight again.

- **Jaw-wiring and stomach stapling.** Jaw-wiring is when someone wires your teeth together so you can't eat any food at all. You can only drink through straws. Stomach stapling is another major operation in which a part of your stomach is stapled together so your stomach can only hold a very small amount of food. If this goes wrong, death may result.

Dieting – a balanced view

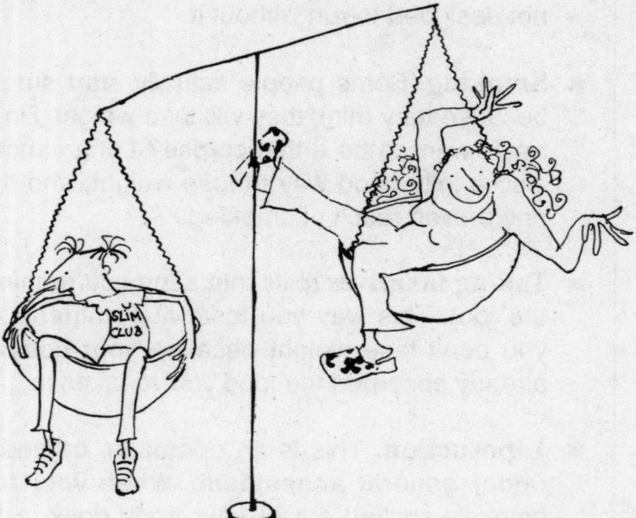

THE PLUS POINTS

- If you can stick to a diet for two weeks or more, you will probably lose weight and you will keep it off as long as you stick to the diet.
- While you are dieting, you may experience a buzz – a feeling of being excited that you might be getting slimmer.
- You will feel smug.
- If you can stay with the diet for a month or so, you will probably be able to buy a smaller clothes' size.

THE MINUS POINTS

Dieting screws up your brain

Your brain – although faster and more complex than the most advanced computer – is a bit slow when it comes to understanding the concept of dieting.

- *You* think you're depriving yourself of food only to get a nice figure.
- *Your brain* thinks you're not eating enough because there's a food shortage.

A food shortage? Oh no! thinks your brain, this means that there's a chance that there'll be less and less food, and I will die! I'm too young to die! I don't want to die! I'm a lovely little brain, kind to animals, and I haven't even taken my GCSEs yet!

I know what I'll do:
I'll burn up those calories much more slowly. This means the food coming in will last longer. The less food, the more slowly I'll burn up those calories. And if the food shortage is over, I'll still burn calories more slowly, just in case it happens again!

And that's not all. I wouldn't be surprised if my owner simply isn't trying hard enough to find food. Just like she doesn't try learning her French vocabulary. I'll make absolutely sure she tries hard to find me food by making her think of nothing else. I'll give her an obsession with food. I'll make pictures of hot, buttered toast and succulent roast chicken come into her mind, so she feels driven to feed me. Feed me! Feed me now!

I'm doing this because I'm feeling desperate. I'm a poor

little brain, and without food, I don't function properly. I can't concentrate if my body is hungry. I feel dizzy and light-headed and irritable. And if my owner keeps on not eating when she's hungry, I won't be able to help her appetite to tell her when she's really hungry and when she isn't. Ever again.

People forget that when they diet, the brain has to diet too, and the effects can be quite serious.

Concentration and metabolism (the rate you burn up your calories) both suffer, and you become obsessed with food. Try this experiment. For one day forbid yourself from sitting on an armchair. No armchairs, or even settees, whatsoever. At school it might be quite easy but when you get home, and everyone else is lounging about, you'll begin to feel jealous. You'll feel deprived. You'll obsess about not being able to sit in armchairs again, you'll make up for lost time. You won't be out of that armchair at all, probably spending more time in that armchair in one day than you would in two.

Conclusion: – DEPRIVATION LEADS TO OBSESSION. DIETING LEADS TO AN OBSESSION WITH FOOD.

Dieting screws up your body

Losing fat isn't as easy as you might think. Here's what really happens to your body when you deprive yourself of food.

1. You lose weight – but not fat. First you will lose fluid, and then you lose lean muscle tissue. Your body is not keen to burn up the fat deposits in case it needs them to make sure you survive this famine it reckons is going on. Only after a considerable period of time does it burn up the fat.

2. You lose strength, because your muscles are getting smaller. You feel weak and light-headed. You don't feel like exercising, and exercising is good for you.

3. You feel permanently hungry. Your body keeps reminding you it needs refuelling. Your stomach rumbles when you don't want it to.

4. You might get constipated.

5. You might get bad breath.

6. If you keep on dieting, your periods may be affected.

7. Your face, rather than looking rounded and pretty, will look drawn and pale.

Dieting screws up your personality

Will your friends really like you more if you go on a diet? Almost certainly not…

1. You will think about little else but your diet. You'll lose interest in your friends' lives, and they will lose interest in you because you'll go on about

dieting all the time. People who only talk about what they're eating and what they're not eating are mega-boring.

2. You will think you're fat. Remember, whatever you focus on, grows. When you diet in an attempt to get slimmer, you're always looking at your body in mirrors to see whether you're losing weight. So you keep focusing on those lumps and bumps. The weird thing about dieting is that as soon as you lose one bump, another appears. I have never met a dieter who has reached her target weight and feels she looks perfect. No one's ever perfect. Dieting is endless.

3. You'll keep asking your friends if you're looking slimmer. They'll get fed up, and will think you're getting vain. As indeed you are. People who are obsessed about the way they look are vain.

4. There's a real risk of starting an eating disorder. Dieting can become dangerously obsessive – you'll find you can't stop doing it, like a train with non-functioning brakes. You'll become more terrified than ever of getting fat. So you'll eat less and less and less…

And that's not all, folks…

After the diet

OK, so you didn't get an eating disorder. You couldn't diet any longer because it was your birthday, your sister's wedding, Christmas, whatever. So you broke your diet and slowly went back to eating as you did before. Then this happens:

1. You replace that lean muscle you lost with fat. The body can't store energy in the form of muscle tissue. So you're flabbier than ever.
2. Your metabolic rate doesn't go back up again all by itself. You carry on burning calories more slowly, so you get fatter more quickly.
3. You make up for lost time by eating as much as you possibly can, eating all those delicious things you dreamed about when you were on a diet but didn't allow yourself. So you get fatter.
4. You hate yourself for getting fatter. You get depressed.
5. When you're depressed, you eat.
6. So you get fatter.
7. You're so desperate, you decide you'd better try another diet.
8. So you end up getting even fatter.

Here's a new scientific discovery: all together now –

DIETING MAKES YOU FAT.

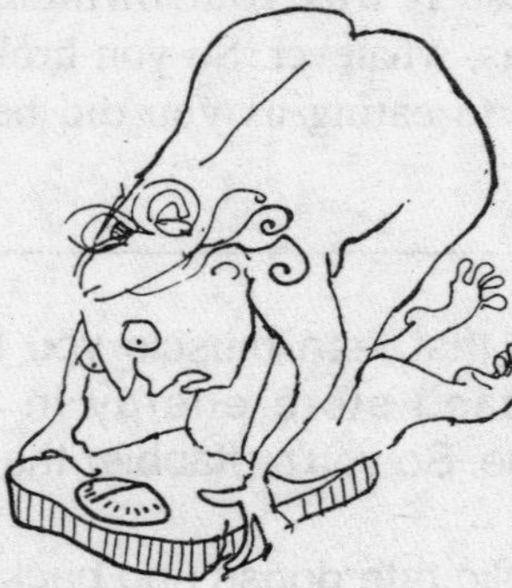

This is the main disadvantage of dieting.

So are you saying that dieting doesn't work?

Yes, I am saying that. Did you know that between 95 per cent and 98 per cent of all dieters, no matter what diet they're on, put all the weight back on after a time? Or let me put it another way. You want a radio/cassette recorder. You buy quite an expensive one. It's hard to get it to work, but it does work for a bit. After six weeks it stops playing. What would you do?

I'd take it back to the shop – ask them to sort it out, or get my money back.

Fine. The right answer. Now try this one. You buy a diet product or go to a slimming club. The diet's hard, but you stick to it for a while and lose weight. Then you can't stick to it any more, and put the weight back on. What would you do?

Think it was my fault.

Wrong! It's the fault of the people who sold you the diet, just like it's the fault of the people who sold you the duff radio. Dieting is a con. It's also a brilliant way to make money.

The scam

You sell a diet.

£

People buy it and you get rich.

£ £

Long term it doesn't work.

£ £ £

The dieters blame themselves for it not working.

£ £ £ £

So they come back and buy the diet again.

£ £ £ £ £

You make even more money.

A lot of the people at any slimming club are people who have rejoined, rather than people who join for the first time, lose all their weight, and never reappear again. It doesn't work like that. Dieting is for life, not just for Christmas. It's a life sentence. And what's the crime? Being fat? Who said being fat was a crime?

You'd be better off believing in Father Christmas and the Tooth Fairy than in the myth that dieting makes you slim.

I heard about dieting from a really early age. There was always talk of it in my house. Even when I was in the infants' my parents wouldn't let me have pudding. I've always been a little plump, and when I was small it didn't bother me, but the older I get, the more it does.

I've been on loads of diets. I've tried Slimfast, I've been to Weight Watchers three times when I was 9, 11 and 12. I've weighed out all my food like they tell you, but I've found it just makes you want to have more. From time to time I starve myself. I've eaten only fat-free food. I've tried diet drinks, I've tried the Combination Diet where you can only eat certain food in combination with other foods.

I keep on starting diets, and losing weight, feeling happy when I can get into smaller clothes, and then when I put the weight back on I feel unhappy with myself. I hate myself when I eat the wrong sort of food. Every week I think I'll cut out chocolate again but just thinking about it, makes me want it more. It's not a good way to live. And I'm as plump as I ever was.
(Janice, 14)

If you diet for two weeks, you can burn up calories up to 20 per cent more slowly.

So if you're really set on getting slim, dieting isn't the answer. It's part of the problem. Look around you. The chances are the bigger women you see are the ones who've spent a lifetime dieting; the ones with OK figures have probably never tampered with their bodies by playing around with their food intake.

There's only one conclusion – dieting is daft.

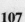

FAT

Chapter 7

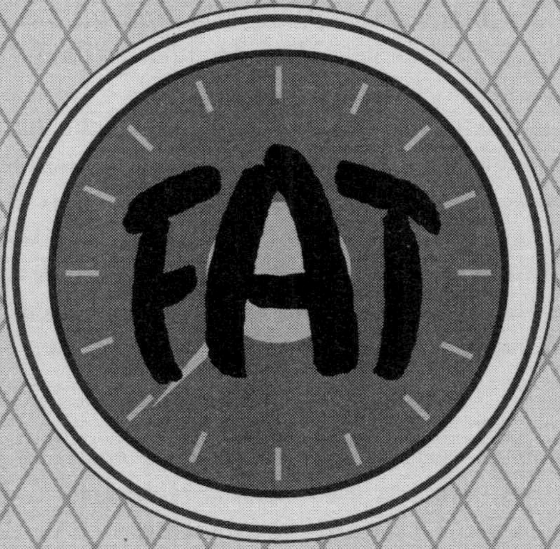

An ABC of eating disorders

Anorexia

What is anorexia?

Anorexia nervosa is an illness that affects the way you think about food and weight. Someone suffering from anorexia believes she is fat when she is not, and she will eat as little as she possibly can in order to lose weight. She may also exercise excessively. Anorexics believe they are fat even when they are painfully thin, and will lie about the amount of food they eat. They become terrified of putting on weight.

If an anorexic loses a great deal of weight, her periods will stop. Her body will go back to its childhood state. Her breasts will stop growing. She may even start to grow a layer of hair on her body for insulation. Her bones may become brittle and she can injure herself easily, as well as being prone to illness. Untreated, anorexia can lead to death. 14 out of 15 anorexia sufferers are female.

I've had anorexia for about two years now. The funny thing was, it wasn't even me who recognized it. It was my mum. But I'll start at the beginning.

I remember getting worked up about the exams at the end of year 8. It was important to me to do well – I had a very clever friend – and I decided I would work as hard as I could. There were books spread out all over my bedroom. I just thought that if I did really well at school people would praise me, and I'd be good at something. I felt I wasn't any good at anything.

And it was about that time I began to eat less and less. Not eating was something else I knew I could be good at, and I thought slim people were successful too. They were popular and got the boys. I didn't go on a diet, so much as just eat less and less, seeing how much I could do without.

I would watch the clock, only allowing myself to eat at certain times. It got so I was watching the clock all the time. I'd put food out so Mum would think I was eating something. The more I lost weight, the fatter I felt, and the more I hated myself. I thought I needed to do more, so I began to exercise, at night and first thing in the morning.

Then Mum realized something was up and she took me to the doctor. He told me to eat three meals a day, so I just said I did. That was all that happened.

So I began to eat even less. On a typical day I would have an apple for breakfast, and then an apple for lunch. In the evening I ate what my mother would give me, but I always made sure I left something on my plate. If I was hungry the only thing I would allow myself was an apple. Eventually my mum insisted I saw the doctor again. I began to get scared. I didn't want him to weigh me. I cried to Mum that I didn't want to go because I didn't want to face up to the problem. It takes me a long time to come forward and speak to people. I'm the sort of person that, if I have a problem, I won't come forward for help.

This time when I went to the doctor, he said my pulse rate was very low, and he made me promise to drink milk. Finally Mum insisted that I get proper treatment. They decided to send me away to a specialist centre for treating eating disorders.

Then my weight loss wasn't my secret any more. We had to tell my Nan and my best friend. Everybody was so shocked. They'd seen me getting thinner, but as my best friend said, she could never imagine anorexia actually happening to someone real, someone she knew.

I felt such a failure. I thought I'd let the whole family down, and that everyone would be better off without me. I was nothing. I had no life. I was very depressed. I loved my family so much but I wished they didn't love me, as it would have made everything so much easier. My mistake was in wanting to be perfect. I can see now my family never wanted me to be perfect – they wanted the old Jane back.

The night before I was sent away was awful. I was scared. I was scared of being away from home, and that night I insisted on sleeping in my mum and dad's room. I cried so much that no one slept. Before I was admitted, I had to go shopping to buy clothes with elasticated waists for when I was going to put weight on. That also frightened me. The idea of putting weight on was a nightmare. Yet I'd got so thin the only clothes that would fit me were children's clothes. Even then, I looked in the mirror and saw a fat person. I hated it when people told me I was thin because I knew they were lying to make me feel better.

All the way to the treatment centre I was crying in the car, and apologizing to my mother. When I checked in I was cold and shivering because I was undernourished. I was given my own bedroom. We had therapy every day. They weighed us every day, and we had to be naked. I had no privacy at all. They watch you in the showers and when you went to the toilet, you had to leave the door open. This was in case you tried to make yourself sick. So you couldn't go to the toilet unless a nurse was there. I found this very degrading.

Of course, they fed me, too. The food seemed never-ending. For the therapy, we had to keep a diary about our feelings towards food, weight, relationships and our moods. Then we discussed what we had written, showed it to a nurse, and shared our feelings in a group. We had to do role plays of situations in our lives that made us nervous. One of the things that I found the hardest was the work we did on body image. As an anorexic I'd grown to hate my body, and saw it as fat and grotesque. What we had to do was take parts of our clothing off, and we had to describe what we saw to the rest of the group. Everyone hated that.

In the end I began to realize I was scared of growing up, both physically and mentally. Yet at the same time I wanted to impress boys. I thought if I was thin boys would automatically fancy me. I learned that I was unsettled and insecure in my friendships too, and not eating seemed like a solution to that.

I was in the treatment centre for five weeks. I could have stayed longer, but I rushed the treatment because I wanted to get home. Then I had to go back again because I realized I wasn't better. By then the funding had run out, so I had to go back as a day patient.

I'm beginning to get better now. I've stopped the lying, and tell people the truth about myself and what I eat. I still find it very hard to eat, and a bad day at school will send my eating haywire. It upsets me when my Nan tries to feed me and I just can't eat. At least I'm going in the right direction now. Sometimes I get very angry when I see anorexia depicted on television, and it's so inaccurate. Shannon on 'Home and Away' was supposed to have anorexia, and she got better in a few weeks. A few weeks. It's been two years for me, and I've still got a long way to go.

(Jane, 14)

Does dieting cause anorexia?

No, but it can trigger it. If a girl has the type of personality that might make her likely to be an anorexic, an episode of dieting might tip her over into the illness. It's a bit like asking whether having an alcoholic drink will turn you into an alcoholic. It will, if you have the tendency to be an alcoholic.

However, some girls get so obsessed with dieting that they have symptoms very similar to true anorexia, hating themselves and their bodies, thinking they're fat when they're not, and refusing to eat. The trouble is, in our society where thinness is considered fashionable, we don't notice when a girl is becoming very thin. People will even congratulate her on losing weight, when they ought to be extremely worried instead. So a lot of anorexics have their illness well established before people realize what is *wrong* with them.

What should you do if you think your friend has got anorexia?

There's always a lot in the newspaper and in magazines about anorexia, and some girls think their friends are anorexic when they might not be. The time to worry is when a friend of yours rarely eats in front of you, throws away her packed lunch, and is getting thinner and thinner. Another clue is that an anorexic will try to hide her weight loss by wearing baggy clothes. A girl who is naturally very thin will be more likely to show off her body by wearing figure-hugging clothes.

But if you really do suspect your friend might be ill, try talking to her first. If she confesses to you that she does have a problem, you must try to get her to talk to a parent, teacher or responsible adult. If she denies she's ill, but you are increasingly convinced she is, talk to your mum or dad, or failing that, a teacher. Anorexics need professional help. If you do have a friend who is suffering from anorexia, don't feel guilty if you can't help her. You wouldn't try to cure your friend by yourself if she had bronchitis – you'd get her off to a doctor double quick. It's the same with anorexia. Sometimes your friend might just be on a diet that's out of control – in that case she'll be more likely to want to talk to you about it.

If your friend isn't a true anorexic but is simply dieting too strictly, you may be able to help. If your friend does have anorexia, there are still ways you can support her.

I knew Jane was getting thinner. Even my parents spoke to me about her, but I didn't want to say anything at first, because I didn't want to hurt her feelings. Then one evening she came to our house for a family meal, and I noticed she only ate one piece of fish and one potato. I began to worry, but still, I held back from saying anything. I didn't want to upset her. When we went back to school at the end of the summer holidays, I could really see how thin she'd become. I was shocked. It was then that Jane told me she was going into the treatment centre for anorexia. She showed me leaflets about the hospital.

Once she'd gone into the hospital, I wrote letters to her about school, so she could keep up with everything. It was a hard time. There was gossip about Jane – some people were seriously concerned, and others seemed just curious. All the time I was very, very worried about her. What if she didn't get better? I felt sort of helpless. I wanted to make her better but I couldn't do anything for her – she was so far away. Then when I thought back over the past few months, I felt guilty. I thought I should have realized when I saw Jane throwing her dinner away. I visited her lots of times and saw her parents. I thought it was important to keep up our friendship.

Now she's back at school it's much better. I'm pleased she seems to be improving, and I still want to be there for her.

(Judith, 15)

At first I started dieting because everyone was doing it. When I say 'dieting', I mean we all ate apples instead of crisps, and went around saying that we were worried about our weight. But I wasn't losing anything. One day I went over to the school canteen and discovered I didn't have quite enough money for a proper lunch. So I thought I'd skip lunch, and that would have the added good effect of helping me to lose weight. I decided I would manage with just one meal a day, and then I'd be bound to get thinner.

If I got hungry, I'd blame myself. I told myself that other people could get by without lunch, and I was just being greedy. The trouble was, I wasn't losing as much weight as I wanted. So I began telling my mum that I'd already eaten at school, and I refused my evening meal. I was eating less and less. Then my friends began to notice. They were beginning to hassle me, going on about why I wasn't eating. They began to get on my nerves. I felt as if I knew what I was doing, and they were interfering, they were even jealous, because they couldn't resist eating, whereas I could. If they invited me to their houses, and I had to eat out of politeness, I really resented it.

In the end, my friends spoke to a teacher about me.

She approached me to have a chat. She told me that it was dangerous, what I was doing. I hadn't thought of it that way before. She told me that if I carried on not eating, my periods would stop, and eventually that might stop me having babies. That shocked me. I've always loved children, and the thought that I might not be able to have any, really scared me. I'd not seen it in that light before. I decided I had to try to eat more. I went to a discussion group at school where different girls talked about their problems with weight, and I heard that I wasn't the only one worried about being fat. It amazed me to think that people who were so pretty and slim had the same negative feelings about themselves as me. We all felt we were monsters, but everybody else felt all the other people looked fine. I still felt fat deep down, but I did begin to eat more, and my weight became normal again.
(Nicola, 17)

Do anorexics make themselves sick?

Not necessarily. Anorexia is an illness when you starve yourself; some, but not all, anorexics, will also eat a large quantity of food and then make themselves sick in order to get rid of it.

Bulimia

What is bulimia?

Bulimia nervosa is the proper name for the eating disorder when you regularly make yourself sick in order to control your weight. Whereas an anorexic is always painfully thin and getting thinner, a bulimic may be normal weight, or even quite large. This means that it's harder to know whether someone is bulimic or not. Bulimics are often very ashamed of what they do. They feel disgust, and are less likely to tell people about their problem, or ask for help – although it is true that Princess Diana told the country about her bulimia on television. But that was only after she'd found a cure for it.

How often do bulimics make themselves sick?

If you have tried making yourself sick once or twice, that doesn't mean you have bulimia, just as someone who tries skipping lunch for a week isn't an anorexic. Someone who is suffering from bulimia will throw up once a day, and then more frequently, sometimes after every meal. It can get harder and harder for a bulimic to get rid of food, and so she will also use laxatives, or sometimes put objects down her throat to make herself sick. This can be highly dangerous, as the object can be swallowed and a major operation might be necessary.

Not only that, but regularly making yourself sick to control weight will wear away the enamel on your teeth, and will result in stomach disorders. Eventually, like anorexia, it can kill you.

When I first read about bulimia in a magazine I was disgusted. Then one day I was coming home on the bus and there were some boys I knew on the bus, and I fancied one of them. His friend came up to me when the top of the bus was empty, and said, 'You fancy my friend, don't you?' I didn't say anything. Then he said, 'Well, he won't go out with you, because you're fat.' I ignored him.

But I was very upset. That night, the boy I fancied rang me and said it wasn't true, and he apologized for what his mate had said. But he didn't ask me out. So it must have been true, I thought. I was too fat. Then I decided I must lose weight. I went into the toilet and stuck my fingers down my throat. It was easier than I thought to make myself sick.

It was also easy for me because my mum works nights. No one was around. I cleared up very carefully, and that was that. I realized I could eat what I wanted if I was sick afterwards, so I did it again the next night.

I felt pleased with myself. It was like, this was my secret. No one else was going to know about it. I did begin to lose weight, and I got a buzz from that. Then one day I had a big lunch at school, so I went to the toilets at school, and threw up there. It was getting easier for me to throw up. I could just think sick, and be sick.

Then I began to throw up after every meal, and every time I ate. I thought that would make me lose weight more quickly. I couldn't sleep at night, I suppose because my body wanted food, and sometimes I even got up in the night and had something to eat, and made myself sick.

The important thing was that nobody should find out. I knew my mum would make a fuss, but at the time she was involved at work. I don't have a dad. Well, I did, but he left us. I was glad because he was violent. To me as well.

Anyway, at school, I was careful too. Because when you make yourself sick, you sort of strain your face and your eyes go all red and watery. So I took face powder to school with me to hide the redness, and also I made a point of eating in front of my friends, so they wouldn't suspect anything. Then if I wanted to be alone to throw up, I'd wait till lessons had started, and then ask if I could be excused.

In the end the bulimia was ruling my life. It took over completely and I just thought about it all the time. Part of me was very scared but the other part just pushed me on. It was like I was punishing myself, and I thought I deserved punishment. Once after I was sick I kept scratching my wrist with my compass until the blood ran. I had to wear long sleeves even though it was summer so nobody could see what I'd done.

Then one day I went to the toilets at school during English. I don't know why but I wasn't being very careful. I didn't notice that one of the toilet doors was shut, and when I came out after being sick there was a girl standing by the hand drier, a girl from the year above me. She asked me if I was all right and I panicked and I was rude to her. I said it was none of her business.

So she reported the incident to the teacher, and the Head of Year spoke to me. I lied to her. I said I hadn't been well. But this teacher knew all about me, about my dad and everything, and she said she'd been noticing I'd been losing weight. She kept probing and in the end I broke down. I thought she was going to be really disgusted with me. Instead she was very sympathetic, and said I should tell my mum.

I wouldn't do that. I knew my mum would be furious. But the teacher explained I would have to tell my mum eventually because I would need to see a doctor. Telling Mum was the hardest thing in the world, and I felt so horrible, especially after all she'd been through with Dad. I thought she would hit me but she just cried. In a way that was worse.

I did go to the doctor, and he made me see a specialist, a psychiatrist at the hospital. It took me six months before I could stop being sick and even now when I feel depressed I want to do it. The psychiatrist made me see that I was trying to control my food because I couldn't control other things that had happened to me in my life, and part of getting better was uncovering some horrible memories. I blamed myself for the bad things that happened to me. I thought I was worthless and so I punished myself.

What I'm learning now is that it's important to respect yourself. If I'd respected myself, I would have never started being sick. I've got a boyfriend now, but not that boy I fancied. I've told him about my bulimia and he doesn't mind. So I'm hoping it won't come back again, ever.

(Karen, 18)

What is the treatment for bulimia?

Very much the same as for anorexia. A specialist will investigate the psychological reasons that lie behind this eating disorder with the aim of gradually getting you to let go of the habit. Sometimes treatment takes place in groups. A cure can take a very long time, and even then, there may be patches in your life when bulimia will recur. Strange as it may seem, the habit of throwing up after you eat can be very addictive, just like drugs and alcohol. Like anorexics, bulimics are terrified of getting fat. For them it's a real phobia, just like you might have a phobia about spiders or heights.

How can I help a friend with bulimia?

You may suspect a friend has bulimia if you regularly hear

her being sick in the toilets, or if a friend or family member tries to drown the sound of whatever she is doing in the bathroom. But a bulimic will only admit to what she is doing when she has reached desperation point. If you suspect a friend is bulimic, you can help by not going on about how fat you or other people are. I'm sure the number of eating disorders would go down if the rest of us stopped worrying about weight, making people with real eating disorders think that it must be the worst thing in the world to be fat. Because it isn't.

Compulsive overeating

Is bingeing an eating disorder?

Again, it depends. All of us pig out occasionally. Most people overeat from time to time. It's quite normal to try to cheer yourself up with chocolate.

But there is an eating disorder called compulsive overeating. This is when a person has no control over the amount of food they eat, and will have vast quantities of food at one sitting, often not caring about what the food is, or what it tastes like. Compulsive overeaters might just eat uncooked flour, or food that has gone off, or anything that's edible, just cramming more and more in. Like a bulimic, they might be very ashamed of what they do, and so they might hide supplies of food in secret places, just like an alcoholic will hide a supply of drink. Elvis Presley almost certainly died of compulsive overeating, consuming well over 55,000 calories a day. (An average man consumes 2,000 to 3,000 calories a day.)

Compulsive overeating can be a very frightening condition. Some compulsive overeaters will have periods of starving themselves, or vomiting, so their weight is controlled. Otherwise, like Elvis Presley, they will get very fat. Compulsive overeaters need professional help too. It's not something you can fight alone.

However, don't confuse a one-off binge with compulsive overeating. If you've had one of those nights when you can't seem to stop going to the fridge or the biscuit tin, you're just like millions of people everywhere. It's when you can't stop overeating that you might have a problem.

Chapter 8

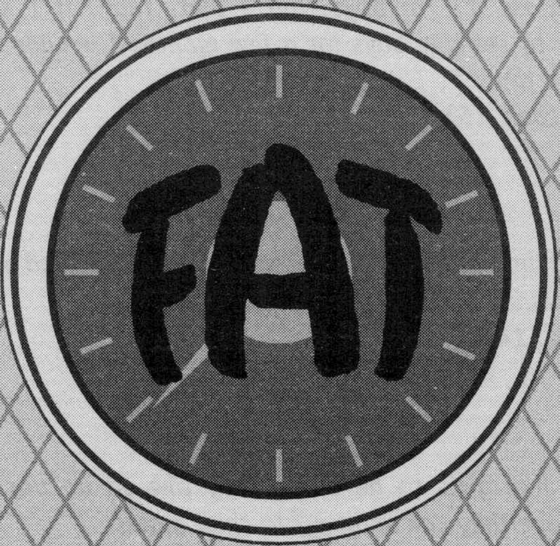

But will he fancy me if I'm fat?

If I know I'm going out in the evening and meeting boys, I starve myself all day. And I don't like to eat in front of lads.
(Jaci, 15)

I suppose it's for boys that I diet. Yeah, if I wasn't going to see any boys for a few months I wouldn't diet all the time.
(Heather, 15)

I wouldn't fancy a fat boy so I can understand why a boy wouldn't fancy me.
(Clare, 14)

Boys like girls to be slim. They like to go out with someone they can show off to their mates.
(Kylie, 13)

I spend ages in front of the mirror before I go out, checking I don't look fat. When I'm actually out, I forget about looking fat.
(Louise, 13)

> *Boys act differently when they're with their friends. On their own, they're not that bad. A boy will only call you fat if he's with his friends.*
> ***(Eilish, 13)***

So is it true? Do you damage your chances with boys if you don't have the perfect figure? Will you die a spinster if you weigh more than nine stone? Do all boys fancy Kate Moss? Would they give up their skateboards, computers and their Manchester United season tickets for a snog with Pamela Anderson? What do boys really want?

Our Fearless Investigator ventures into the locker room to ask the lads about girls and weight, and receives some unexpected replies…

FEARLESS INVESTIGATOR:
Do you fancy girls who are overweight?

Andy: I don't fancy girls who are excessively fat. Or embarrassingly fat. I don't fancy Jo Brand.

Dave: Yeah, if they're too fat it affects their face as well.

Steve: Girls who are just a bit overweight try harder – you know – they tend to be good to have a laugh with. They're nicer.

Colin: It matters more if you don't know a girl – then you look at her figure. But if she's someone you know, like at school, you don't notice what size she is.

Steve: Being slim is only one factor.

FEARLESS INVESTIGATOR:
So what do you fancy in a girl?

Andy: Her face.

Neil: Hair. Hair's important.

Keith: Her eyes.

Neil: Yeah.

FEARLESS INVESTIGATOR:
If you fancied a girl, and she was fat enough for your friends to mention it to you, would you still ask her out?

Steve: Yes, definitely.

Andy: I might think twice about it, but I'd ask her out in the end.

Colin: Yeah. You wouldn't want to pass up on a girlfriend, just because your mates were laughing. That's sad. Your mates are probably jealous.

Keith: If you really like her you don't care what your friends think.

FEARLESS INVESTIGATOR:
Do you fancy really thin girls, the supermodel waifs?

Colin: No way!

Andy: Like Jodie Kidd? No, she's way too thin. Come to think of it, there's this skeleton in the Biology lab. I quite fancy her.

Dave: Kate Moss has got a nice face but her body is too thin.

Neil: Yeah. She's very pretty but she needs to put on some weight.

FEARLESS INVESTIGATOR:
Can you describe your ideal shape for a girl?

Andy: Yeah. She's got to have a nice, round figure, with – erm –

Colin: A bum and boobs.

Andy: Yeah, that's it.

Keith: And no bones sticking out anywhere.

Dave: Except cheekbones.

Steve: And you want a girl to go in at the waist.

FEARLESS INVESTIGATOR:
Like Pamela Anderson?

Andy: No, not her. She's got a horrible skin texture.

Neil: She's plastic, like a Barbie doll.

Keith: She's a bimbo.

Dave: I wouldn't say no.

FEARLESS INVESTIGATOR:
What do you think of girls who diet?

Neil: My sister is really skinny but she reckons she's fat. She eats salads all the time. She's stupid. She's only fourteen. I think she just does it to seem older.

Steve: Yeah, my older sister diets. She's 20. She goes to Weight Watchers. When she stops going, she puts all the weight she's lost back on. It's pointless.

Andy: It's weird. Girls diet and boys don't. But girls aren't fatter than boys.

Neil: All the girls I know are permanently on diets.

Andy: It's dangerous. They might get anorexia.

Colin: Why is it that all the girls who go on diets are never fat in the first place?

Steve: It's mad. All the girls want to lose weight but the boys aren't bothered.

Keith: I find it annoying, the way girls are always on about what they should and shouldn't be eating. My last girlfriend was permanently paranoid. It's boring.

Colin: I like a girl who's happy with herself – who *isn't* obsessed and talking about her weight all the time.

Andy: Yeah.

Steve: I agree with that. Once you're going out with someone, you want to enjoy yourself. You don't want to have her worrying about putting on weight all the time. If she comes over like *she* thinks she's good-looking, you end up fancying her more.

Andy: As you get older, personality counts more, anyway.

FEARLESS INVESTIGATOR:
Do you ever call your sisters – or other girls – fat?

Steve: Yeah, but I'm just mucking around.

Neil: You do at primary school, just to be one of the crowd. I remember we used to call this girl 'pudding'. She didn't seem to be bothered, though.

Colin: You wouldn't call a girl fat if you really thought she was.

FEARLESS INVESTIGATOR:
Do any of you worry about being fat?

Dave: No.

Andy: No.

Colin: But it's getting worse. There's all these images of men now, male models and groups like Boyzone. You feel you've got to compete with all of them.

Andy: Speak for yourself. I reckon they've got to compete with me.

(Andy, Dave, Neil, Colin, Keith and Steve are all 15 or 16 – and all very fanciable! And not all thin!)

WHO IS THE WOMAN THAT TEENAGE BOYS FANCY MOST? (Try to guess.)

Answer:
Marilyn Monroe: 'she makes you tingle…', sez Steve.
Marilyn was an Amerian size 12 (British size 16).

90 per cent of the world's cultures think fat hips and fat thighs are sexy.

Don't kid yourself that if you're wafer-thin the boys will be knocking passers-by down in their attempts to get to you. They won't. They'll be after the girls with real female bodies – with boobs and bums.

If they can get them. Just like real girls aren't all thin, real boys aren't perfect either. *They* also worry about their appearance, although it's true they're less likely to worry about their weight. If they do weigh themselves, it's usually in the hope they've put some weight on. Boys like to be big. Most boys – like you – want a girlfriend who likes them. That's the biggest turn on there is. Boys choose girlfriends for a variety of different reasons, but I've never seen the boy yet who goes round parties and discos with a tape measure and scales, checking out the vital statistics of the opposite sex.

What matters in pulling boys is your charisma – and you get that from self-confidence.

What do boys worry about?

Out of a random sample of 28 boys:

9 worried about their hair. Is it too curly? Too short? Too long? Is it the wrong colour? Does the dandruff show?

8 worried about their height. They all wanted to be taller. No boy wants to be short. They all like to look older than they are.

3 worried about spots. The genuine Biactol boys.

3 worried about their build. Get out those muscle expanders, lads!

5 didn't worry about anything. Bliss!

28 worried about whether their team was going to avoid relegation this season.

Not one worried about weight.

As far as boys go, there's a good saying: *Those that mind don't matter, and those that matter, don't mind.* Any boy who is only interested in the appearance of your figure isn't interested in you anyway. You're only a trophy girlfriend, someone he can show off to his mates. No one wants to be treated as an object. And the boy who tries to tell you to lose weight, or to shape up to his idea of what a girl should look like, is extremely immature and too bossy. Drop him quick. Any boy worth having will allow you to make decisions about your figure, and value you for more than your body – although he'll value your body too. Just like you value his!

And why spend the whole of your friend's birthday party checking out your own figure when you could be checking out the gorgeous hunk in the corner who looks like Shane from *Home and Away*? Girls who worry too much about their appearance are in danger of falling in love with themselves rather than a boy. Don't worry about what the boys think of you – instead, worry about what you think about the boys.

Fat and sex

My mum worries that I'll go too far with my boyfriend if she leaves us alone in the house. But I've told her – I'd never take my clothes off in front of Pete. I'm so embarrassed about my stomach. And I'd never let him see me with the lights on.
(Tracy, 16)

It's true that females have wide hips for having babies, and breasts for feeding them with. But that's not all boobs and hips are for. They're also meant to attract the opposite sex, so you can grow a baby in the first place.

Boys find curves attractive. They're a turn-on. If you don't believe that, go to your local newsagent, go to the magazine section, stand up very, very tall, now – on to your tiptoes – and reach down one of those naughty magazines from the top shelf. Have a look at the pin-ups. Are they flat-chested? If they turned sideways, would they disappear?

These are the women that men fantasize about – not the tiny models who wear skinny rib jumpers in teen magazines. Sex is all about feeling people, about sensation. You don't make a baby by looking at someone. What boys enjoy about snogging and what comes after is the *feel* of a girl – and girls who are overweight are every bit as nice to feel as average weight girls; some might even say that they're nicer. Boys like girls because they're cuddly, not because their stomachs are like a washboard.

And the last thing you want during a passionate embrace is the sound of your stomach rumbling because you skipped tea as you didn't want to look fat.

The not-very-thin Girl's Guide to flirting

1. Don't dress in dowdy colours so no one will notice your body. If you do that, no one will notice *you*. Wear a splash of colour, or something attention-drawing. Look like you mean business.

2. If you think make-up suits you, go for it. Take

your hard-earned pocket money down to Boots, and spend, spend, spend. Invest in some snog-proof lippie, and some mascara so you can flash those lashes.

3. And use your eyes. Eyes speak louder than anything. At the party look at the boy you fancy, then look away as if you didn't mean it. Make sure he sees you doing it. Intrigue him.

4. Wear perfume. A whiff of something nice as you pass by also has an effect.

5. Smile. A smile is the most powerful love potion there is. Everyone is attracted to people who smile. They look like they might be fun to get to know.

6. Let him know you like him. Go up and talk to him, and if you have enough confidence, you can always ask him out. There's no law against it.

7. Once in conversation with him, look as if you're interested in what he's saying. Unless, of course, you realize that you've just hooked the Amateur Bore of the Year and you'll scream if he goes on about fly-fishing another moment longer.

8. Talk back. Don't be a Yes girl. Show him you've got a mind of your own as well as a body – and both are extra-special.

9. Don't keep pulling in your stomach or slumping your shoulders so he won't see you're a 36B.

Be proud of your natural assets. (Boys like natural assets! They're fascinated by boobs – make sure he knows you've got some!) Besides, if you look distracted worrying about your figure, he'll think he's boring you.

10. Don't give the impression you're too desperate. Play it cool. *You* know he'll be lucky to get you; let *him* realize he'll be lucky to get you, too.

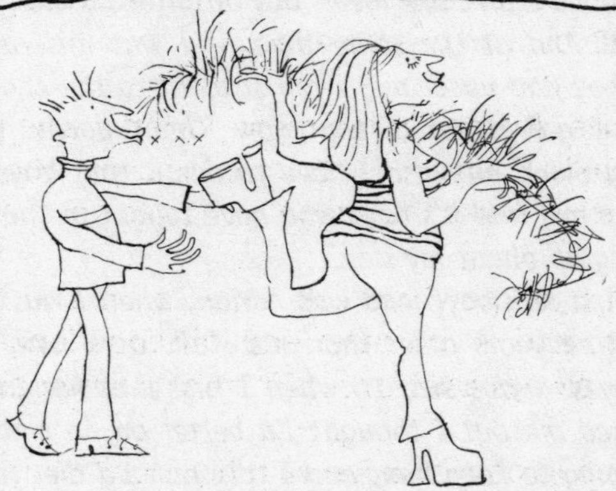

Thought for the day . . . Thought for the day

. . . Thought for the

Nature intended that different boys should fancy different girls – we weren't all meant to fancy the same person. Imagine the mass murder that would take place if we did. Even if you haven't met the boy who fancies you yet, he's out there somewhere. So you've got to keep looking...

. . . Thought for the
Thought for the day . . . Thought for the day

True romance

Adele is 17 years old, 10st 4lb and size 12 'but I can easily slip in to a size 14' – and 5' 4" tall. She's taking A-levels and hopes to study English at university…

When I was younger I was insecure around boys because of my weight. I equated fat with being ugly. So if someone didn't like me – boy or girl – I'd blame it on my fat. And at the same time, if I was miserable, or some boy had upset me, I ran straight to the chocolate. But I've grown out of that now. That's partly just me getting older, but also I have to admit that boys mean a lot to me, and it's boys who have taught me not to be so hung up about my size.

My first real boyfriend was Adrian, when I was 15. He was three years older than me. Tall, dark hair, bright blue eyes. I was size 16 when I first met Adrian. After he asked me out I thought I'd better go on a diet if I was going to keep him, and I told him I'd diet for him. He turned round and told me not to lose weight. He said I was beautiful just as I was, and I'd look horrible slimmer. That made me feel a lot more confident about my weight, as all my friends fancied Adrian like mad, and he fancied me, and they were all size 10s.

So that was fine, until our relationship started to turn more physical. I reckoned Adrian had only been nice about my weight because he'd only seen me with my clothes on. As soon as he saw the real me, it would be horrendous. Bye, bye Adrian! In fact, the opposite happened. It was like, he was completely in awe of me. At first I was nervous – the lights had to be off. But I didn't need to be. After Adrian and I split up, I had some other not-very-serious boyfriends. I have to say that my size has never stopped boys being attracted to me. Then Paul came along. He was a real looker. He worked out at the gym – he was blond and blue-eyed, with a really cheeky grin. I couldn't believe he'd want to go out with me. But he did. If I went on about my weight to Paul, he'd get dead angry. He couldn't understand why I was so self-conscious about my body. He was really good to me, complimenting me a lot about how I looked, building up my confidence. He made comments about my body that made me see there was nothing wrong with me. He'd say, why have less of Adele, if you can have more of Adele? He told me that women are meant to be soft and rounded. We're still good friends now, even though we drifted apart after a time.

Looking back, Paul was very important to me. He made a big difference to my self-image. If you're the kind of girl who worries about weight because you want to have a boyfriend, it takes a boy to break that spell.

Although I didn't go out with Barry for long, he's worth mentioning. I met him at a party. When he picked me up, he said he fancied me most because I had the best figure of all the girls there – he said I was a woman, and all the other girls looked like boys. They had no shape.

Now I'm going out with Ian. He's the same age as me. That worried me at first, because my other boyfriends had always been a little bit older, and I thought a younger boy would be more influenced by what his friends thought, and wouldn't make independent judgements. I was wrong. Hooray!

I met Ian at a party at a friend's house when his parents were away. A crowd of us stayed all the night. I fancied Ian but it didn't cross my mind to do anything about it. In the morning I looked a wreck. I was wearing a grotty T-shirt, my hair was back, and I'd scrubbed off all my make-up. He says now that he's never seen me look as beautiful as I did then. He kept looking across at me and to be honest, I thought there must be something wrong with me. But then he followed me to the kitchen, and told me he really liked me. I thought he was probably drunk, and it was only when he asked me out for a drink the following Sunday, I discovered he was teetotal!

Then Ian sent me a letter, saying he was too shy to say what he felt, and he would prefer to write it. In the letter he said he was scared of me rejecting him – this dead good-looking captain of the school football and basketball teams – and there I was thinking he couldn't really like me.

Bit by bit we spent more and more time together. It became quite clear that Ian had no problem at all with my size – it was more like the opposite was true. It was an advantage. I began to think maybe all these guys are telling the truth after all. When we went to Alton Towers with a crowd of friends and I went on the scary rides with him I wasted my money. I wasn't scared at all. Ian was with me.

We've been going out for quite some time now. This is a much more mature relationship, not based so much on each other's appearance. We have had our arguments, but we've made them up. Like a lot of boys, if he's depressed about something, he'll bottle it up and go all quiet, and then there's me thinking I've done something. I seem to need quite a lot of reassurance that he still loves me – I think this is probably partly caused by my weight, but that feeling is getting smaller all the time.

Also I can eat with Ian. He took me out to dinner to a Chinese restaurant, and I ate whatever I wanted. To someone who doesn't worry about weight, that might sound odd. But at the beginning of our relationship I wouldn't eat in front of him. I'd rather starve. There was just something about eating in front of a boy. He noticed I wasn't eating when he knew I must be hungry, and he asked me what on earth I was doing? So now I know I can eat freely with him.

I wish I could shout to all the girls who think being overweight will stop them getting boyfriends – IT'S NOT TRUE!

In fact, in my case, I reckon it's been a deciding factor. My weight's been a plus – in every sense.

(Adele, 17)

Chapter 9

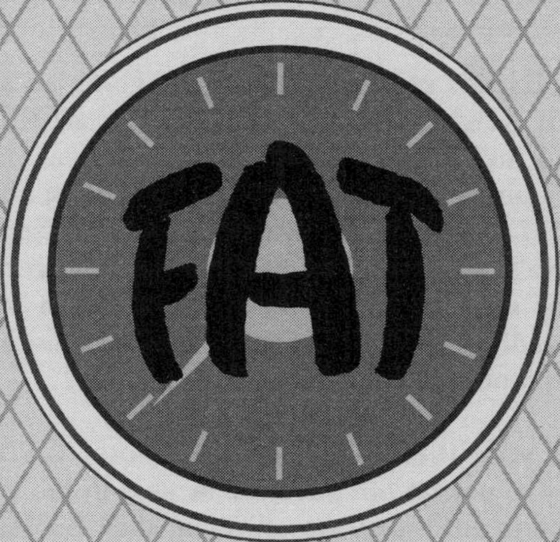

Weigh it up

The weigh it up quiz

If you're beginning to feel more confident now about your weight, try this quiz. Here are five problem page letters, and beneath each are three possible replies. Here's your chance to be an agony aunt. You must choose the correct reply from the three alternatives for each letter. Can you identify the correct ones?

1. My friends at school are always going on about their weight. The trouble is, they're all thinner than me! When we get changed for swimming they pinch their waists and say, 'Look at all that fat!' I can't see any. But it makes me feel as if there's something wrong with me. And recently I've noticed that my friends seem to be excluding me. Do you think if I went on a diet they would like me more?

a) Tell your friends that they're idiots. Tell them they're not fat but severely lacking in the brains department if they go on about their bodies like that. Say that you're much better off than they are as you're not bothered about the way you look. With friends like that, who needs enemies? Treat yourself to a large box of choccies and don't share them with your friends.

b) You know that dieting would only make you more hung up about your weight. From the sound of things, it seems that you might not have a great deal in common with these friends. In your letter you come across as sensitive; I don't think your friends can be very sensitive if they make remarks which hurt you. Time, I think, to investigate other people in your class to see if there is anyone you like more. Remember too, that lots of us blame our fat for things that go wrong in our lives. But it's not the fat's fault! Leave your poor old body alone – it does the best it can for you.

c) Yes, lose some weight. Obviously losing weight is important in your circle of friends, and if you want to fit in with everybody else, you must do as everyone else does. Or even if you don't diet, pretend you're dieting. That way these girls will think that you are like them. Perhaps they'll start being nicer to you then. I hope so. Having good friends is one of the most important things, and it's worth doing anything in order to keep them.

2. My problem is not that I'm fat, but that I'm a beanpole. I've always been skinny since I was a kid. I know it's because I take after my dad – he's 6' 4" and as thin as a rake. I'm 15, and I don't need to wear a bra, and at 5' 8" I tower above most of the boys in my class. I feel so embarrassed about my body. I'm really jealous of the plump girls in my class with real boobs and everything, and they're all dieting! It's mad. But what can I do? I want to put on weight, but nothing seems to work. Help!

a) Lucky ol' you. You have a figure that the rest of us would kill for. Go to your local model agency and get assessed for your modelling potential. Ultra-thin people are in great demand to show today's fashions to advantage. If it turns out that your flat chest is a problem, you can always have silicone implants in your breasts when you are older. Both Pamela Anderson and Paula Yates have had them. Meanwhile, make the other girls in your class jealous by wearing tiny skinny ribs and dead tight jeans. Enjoy yourself!

b) Do you really eat as much as you could? Drink as much full fat milk as possible, eat plenty of bread and butter with your meals, and have frequent snacks – chocolate and peanuts are particularly high in calories. Don't move about too much in case you burn up too much energy. Invest in a Wonderbra which will make the most of whatever breasts you've got. Fry most of your food and suck sweets during lessons. That should make a difference. Knowing you are bigger should help you to overcome your embarrassment.

c) It's always difficult when you don't look the same as everyone else, whether it's because you're overweight or underweight. You feel as if everyone notices you all the time and sees you as different. In fact, that's not true. Most girls of your age are self-conscious about some aspect of their body, just as you are, and they're so worried about themselves they don't notice you! Or they may even be jealous. The best way to come to terms with your figure is to treat yourself to clothes that help you make the most of your appearance, and turn your height and slenderness into assets. If you think you look good, you'll feel more confident, which is what it's all about.

3. There is a gang of girls in our class who keep tormenting me. They follow me about in between lessons and whisper insults: they call me a fat cow, and worse things. It is true I'm three stone overweight, and I can't bear it when people comment about my size. These girls left a note in my locker saying that everyone hated me because I was fat. Or they'll pass me at dinner, and talk to each other about how much I'm eating, and joke that the chair will collapse. Sometimes I pretend to my mum that I'm ill so I can get off going to school. Don't tell me to tell her what's going on because she's fat too, and it might hurt her feelings. Also she's going through a divorce with my dad at the moment. I only want to stop these girls, but I'm really scared of them. Life isn't worth living any more.

a) These girls are bullying you. They must be stopped at once. Bullying is cruel, and no one should have to put up with it. It is not your fault that you are bullied, but it is the fault of these girls. You have nothing to be ashamed of at all. You can't hope to stop the bullying on your own. You need to speak to someone urgently. Since the bullying is taking place in school, you could talk to a teacher. Perhaps she might feel that your mother should know. I think your mother would be even more upset if she knew you were hiding your distress from her. Write down the things the girls say, with the places and times, as the teacher will need this as evidence.

b) Do you have any other friends? If you do, tell them

about what is happening to you. If some of your friends are boys, all the better. Assemble a gang of you, and the next time these girls comment about your weight, get your gang to have a go at them. Even if this ends in a fight, it doesn't matter. You can only fight violence with violence. These girls' comments are violent, and they all deserve a good thumping. Only if they're scared of you will they stop calling you names. Then they might even ask you to join their gang, and you'll certainly be safe from any more attacks.

c) I can see why you don't want to tell your mother what's been happening. She has enough on her plate. These girls are clearly very frightening, and the best thing is to try to avoid going anywhere near them. You were wise to take time off school, and as long as you catch up with the work you've missed, you should do this again. If they wait for you in the canteen, take sandwiches and have your lunch somewhere else. It might also help if you were to lose some weight. Then the girls would not be able to call you fat any more. Till then, wear clothes that disguise your figure.

4. Help! I'm addicted to chocolate. I can't seem to pass a newsagent without going in and getting a bar. If I'm miserable, or even if I want to celebrate, I hit the chocolate. I reckon that on a bad week I can have about fifteen bars. I've read articles in magazines about too much chocolate being bad for you, and I'm worried I'll get fat or ill. Should I try to ration myself? And if I do, will it work? I think I must be the first chocoholic.

a) No; you can find chocolate addicts everywhere. It's very common for girls and women to enjoy eating chocolate. Interestingly, men aren't so bothered about it. Some medical experts think there are substances in chocolate that affect the mood of certain women, and give them a 'high'. Chocolate can produce an effect not unlike falling in love! Some girls are more affected by this than others. Luckily, craving chocolate is not dangerous, even if it's not very good for you. If you can cut your intake down to one bar a day, or a bit less, you'll have no problem. And forgive yourself if on a bad day, you have more.

b) Chocoholism is just like alcoholism. Beware! If your addiction gets worse, you will end up spending all your pocket money, or wages from your newsround, on chocolate. You will stash chocolate away in secret places, under your baby sister's cot, in your pencil case, behind the cistern in the lavatory. Eventually your parents will find out and give you an ultimatum – it's chocolate or them. Powerless to resist the chocolate, you will leave home and end your days sleeping on a park bench covered with Galaxy wrappers. Get yourself into a good recovery programme now. There's no time to be lost!

c) Be gentle on yourself. A little of what you fancy always does you good. Therefore it stands to reason that a lot of what you fancy does you even more good. Fifteen bars of chocolate a week is nothing. Don't risk depriving yourself of something that you so obviously need. Make sure you always have a bar to hand. Did you know you can get bread with chocolate inside, chocolate spread and even chocolate body paste? Cover your arms with this and during lessons you can give yourself a quick fix. Eating chocolate is one of the greatest pleasures a woman can have. Go for it.

5. **Last week I went to the doctor with a nasty cough. It turned out I had a chest infection and he gave me some medicine. As I was getting my top back on, he said to me and my mum that I was a chubby girl and I ought to think about losing some weight. I was very upset and even though I hadn't thought of dieting before, I think I should now. I'm 4' 11" and weigh 10 stone 8 lbs.**

a) If the doctor says you should lose weight, you must lose weight. Either make another appointment to see him and ask him to put you on a diet, or join one of the many slimming clubs in your town. Perhaps the doctor thought your chest infection was made worse by your excess weight. It would be very foolish to ignore anything a doctor says.

b) Your doctor had no right to comment on your weight. You only asked him to help cure your chest infection. At your weight you are not significantly obese, and provided you exercise regularly and eat healthily, you have nothing to worry about. Dieting will only make you fatter in the long run. Doctors are occasionally tactless and ill-informed about weight matters. On this occasion you can safely ignore your doctor's comments.

c) This is outrageous! The doctor was speaking completely out of turn. See your parents' solicitor, and seriously consider taking legal action. If you dieted and contracted an eating disorder, the doctor would be legally responsible. With a bit of luck, you could get him struck off the medical register. For the sake of all the other girls who will pass through his hands, I'd take action now.

The right answers

1. b) Innocent but naïve comments from other girls can have a bad effect on others. In this case, it's best for the writer to find new friends. Confronting them aggressively will only turn the friends into enemies, while dieting to please them will only make them think that the writer doesn't have a mind of her own.

2. c) It can be just as painful to be too thin as it is to be too fat. Both fat and thin girls need to develop their confidence and make the most of themselves. And if you are flat-chested, remember that silicone implants can go wrong. They are bags of gel that a surgeon inserts in your boobs during a major operation. Only for the foolhardy and desperate! Overeating – and especially overeating fatty foods – is bad for everyone, fat and thin alike.

3. a) Bullying is a serious offence, and if it takes place in school, the school will deal with it. Don't try to handle it yourself, and don't just sit there hoping it will go away. No one, but no one, ought to put up with cruelty from others.

4. a) Yes, chocolate cravings are very common. Excuse me while I just have a bite of my Mars bar…

5. b) The doctor is not always right. Doctors who trained a long time ago and are not up-to-date with the latest research about dieting and its bad effects on people, may accidentally give the wrong advice. These days many doctors are rushed off their feet and don't have the time to read the papers that they should. Doctors and nurses are only human and make mistakes. Forgive them, and get on with your own life!

How did you score?

If you selected all five correct answers...

Well done. Not only are you completely sane and sorted about weight issues, but you can think about a career as an agony aunt.

If you selected three or four right answers...

You're getting there. Have the confidence to remember that size isn't really important, not in the long run. We all have the right to live our lives free from unwanted interference.

If you selected two or fewer right answers...

You obviously turned straight to this page and haven't read the rest of the book. Now start from Chapter 1...

Chapter 10

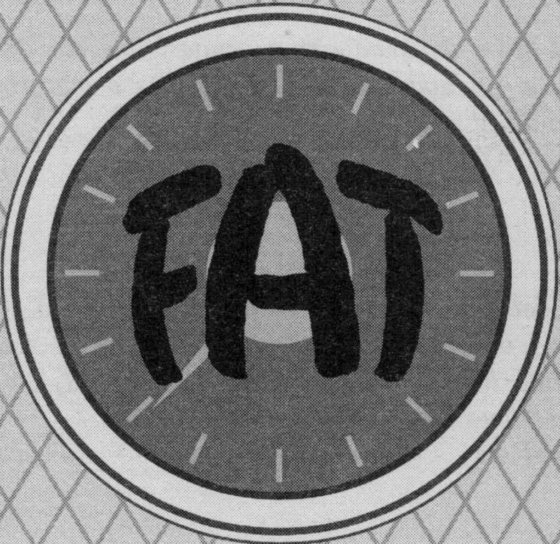

The confidence trick

Looking good

You can be any size and look good. If you think you look good, other people will think so too. Confidence is rather like the common cold – it's infectious. So what obstacles are there for bigger girls who want to look good?

I hate going shopping with my mates. They can fit in all the size 10s and I'm a 14. I feel like a monster. I'm embarrassed in the changing rooms.
(Mary, 14)

I can get into a 12, or sometimes it has to be a 14. But when I do, the clothes look all wrong on me. The material clings and I look fatter than I really am. And the necklines are too low – things like that.
(Rachel, 13)

I'm between a size 16 and 18. I just can't go shopping in the same places my friends go shopping, or if I do, all that fits me is the jewellery. There isn't anything in my size in the chain stores I go to.
(Jessica, 14)

I like to be fashionable and I look in the magazines to see what's in. But the fashions are really only for tiny

girls. I reckon 90 per cent of us are just left out.
(Sian, 15)

It's true that it still isn't easy to be 14 years old and size 14. It's true that most manufacturers of clothes for teenagers (and even older women) aren't providing larger sizes. Some chain stores admit that they buy clothes on a 2-2-1 ratio: that means they buy two size 10s, two size 12s, and one size 14 in each new style. Woe betide you if you are size 16. Until recently, you did not officially exist and even now you can struggle to find fashionable clothes in anything above a size 14. Clothes shops say this is because there isn't a demand for bigger sizes. This would suggest that anyone over size 14 goes around naked. But I've yet to see numbers of nude women strolling around Britain's shopping centres. Someone, somewhere isn't telling the truth.

But let's get real. The chain stores mass produce clothes, and so if you have a figure which is an original shape, it's quite likely mass-produced clothes won't suit you. They're made to suit Miss Normal's figure. Miss Normal is a figment of their imagination – all bodies are differently shaped. So don't feel as if you're a misfit if clothes don't fit you or suit you. The clothes are the misfits, not you. It's the clothes's job to fit you, not the other way round.

So what do you do if you want to look good in a larger size?

1. Don't hide your body in shroud-like baggy clothes. You will only end up looking like a sack of potatoes, or as if you have something to hide. Get clothes that fit you properly.

2. Don't copy clothes for thin girls and expect them to suit you. Baby doll dresses look strange on a girl with a fully-developed figure.

3. Go wild with accessories. Get kooky hats, scarves, chunky jewellery – have fun and look as if you're having fun.

4. Check out the stores where there are cool clothes in larger sizes. Evans have been providing larger sizes for years, but highly recommended are Rogers and Rogers, and for those of you with the cash to spare, Dawn French and Helen Teague's 16/47 – an outlet for glam large size clothes reminding us of the fact that *47 per cent of women are size 16 or over* – a fact which should help you feel more normal.

5. Also shop at the chain stores which try to provide large size ranges. Recommended are River Island's plus sizes, Marks and Spencers (they're getting more fashionable by the day), Warehouse and Etam Plus. There are other stores too.

6. Be creative. Abandon the High Street, and visit some of the New Age-y shops for floaty skirts and tie-dyed T-shirts. Or tie-dye your own. Create a style that is uniquely you.

7. Get *YES!* magazine, which although not aimed exclusively at teenagers, has pages and pages of fashion spreads, all in larger sizes, with

larger models. The mag also lists suppliers of larger clothes all over the country.

8. Take a course in fashion design and be the first person to open up a store especially for 13-18s who need more realistic sizes. It's bound to happen one day.

And remember – it's boring to be little Miss Average – aim to look different.

I'm well over size 16 and I always have been. I've always been this size. I don't overeat. It's just that I put on weight very, very easily. I won't diet. I've seen girls at school become obsessed with dieting and become dangerously thin.

I love clothes. I'm happy that it's no longer a stigma to

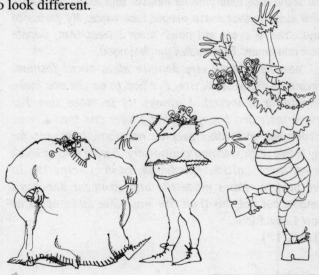

shop at places like Evans. Me and my mum go there and we try absolutely everything on. In our town, the plus-size shops are trendy places to be seen in – so many new ones have opened up recently. It's a growing market, if you'll pardon the pun. The styles are loads better these days. We don't have to camouflage our size any more – we can wear bright colours and be seen.

My current favourite dress is ankle length and it's in a pale grey Lycra-ish material from 16/47. I love it because it's high-waisted, floaty and romantic. I've also got some nice embroidered blouses and loads of T-shirts with slogans that make people look twice. My favourite says, 'You're a big girl now'. When I wear that, people look and smile. That makes me feel good.

I now have some very definite ideas about fashion. Because I'm not stock size, I've had to go out and make something of myself. I always try to make sure I'm comfortable and happy in what I wear and then I know I can cope with other people's reactions. Last year, for my Nan's 50th wedding anniversary, I wore a long black velvet dress, lipstick, foundation, earrings – the lot. In the past my Nan's made the odd comment about my weight, but not this time. She was quite taken aback at how I could look.

(Leah, 17)

Feeling good

You are what you eat

No, it's all right. If you eat too many carrots you won't turn orange and develop a rough skin. Nor will you start saying 'What's Up, Doc?' or be able to see in the dark. But what you eat does play a big part in how you feel.

Should I cut out all junk food, then?

Not all of it. Otherwise you won't be able to lead a normal lifestyle. If your mates are going for burger and chips, you don't want to sit outside the restaurant virtuously nibbling at your organic wholefood hi-energy fat-free sandwich. But a diet based on too much fatty or sugary foods will make you feel cloggy and heavy, whatever size you are. Don't overdo the junk.

So I must try to eat loads of fruit and vegetables.

Too much fruit, and you'll be permanently on the loo. Two or three pieces a day is fine. And try to have a helping or two of veggies every day. That can include baked potatoes, and raw vegetables: they're filling and full of vitamins. Oh, and there's nothing magic about salad. Did you know that there's very little nutrition in a lettuce leaf? Live on lettuces alone, and you'll suffer from malnutrition.

What should I eat if I want to feel good?

Three meals a day – your body needs regular food if it's going to function properly. Different sorts of food – plenty of brown bread, pasta, rice, potatoes, some fish and meat, beans, fruit, veg and dairy products too. If you eat a wide range of food regularly, you'll feel great. See the healthy eating triangle in Chapter 5.

Shall I make out my own diet based on healthy eating?

No. Any inflexible eating plan means you're bound to deviate from it. Just relax about food. Don't obsess about it. Enjoy what you eat, then go off and do something more interesting.

I'm sport-crazy. I play netball, badminton, hockey, squash and compete in athletics. At one time I was training for the pentathlon. My coach told me I had to watch what I ate. He told me to keep a food diary, and he would check my nutrition level.

My official lunch was something like two apples, a banana, a cheese sandwich, a wheat health bar and a tangerine. My coach hoped I would lose weight because in athletics extra weight can slow you down. I was also given lots of extra exercises to do.

I kept to this diet for a while, but then I was so hungry at school that when no one was around, I went crazy and ate loads and loads of chocolate. I'd eat up to four chocolate bars with my lunch. Then at home I'd exercise furiously in order to get rid of it. Dieting like that does your head in.

It was taking over my life – all that training and having to watch every mouthful I ate. Then I got injured – I tore a ligament. That enforced break made me realize that I wasn't handling the pressure. I just couldn't hack it any more. I decided to give up athletics as the price was too high. I just wasn't prepared to pay it. Looking back, I can see that decision was the best one I'd ever made.

Now I eat much more sensibly. I make sure I'm not hungry, then I'm not tempted to fill myself with chocolate. I learned that the idea of not being allowed to eat something made you want to eat it. I'd never diet again.

Even though I've given up athletics, I still play lots of sport as I really enjoy it. My parents are PE teachers and it's a kind of family thing with us. Right now I play lots of squash, and look forward to matches. It's much better when sport is for enjoyment. Being physically active helps me take a sane attitude to my body. I don't obsess about my appearance – I like my body because it works for me.

(Laura, 15)

Fit for life

Rather than staring at your body in the mirror wishing it was all different, get out and use it. Exercise is the best way to feel good, do yourself good, and even improve your mood. Exercise releases special chemicals into your blood stream which give you a 'high', and put you in a positive frame of mind. There's also mounting evidence to show that exercise is every bit as important as healthy eating, and that fit people even live longer too.

Whatever size you are, you should think about taking regular exercise.

Yes, but the problem with most forms of exercise is that you have to take your clothes off. I like swimming but I hate having to walk across to the pool and everyone seeing my flabby bits. And it's even worse on the beach.

True. Try to cheer yourself up with the thought that most other people are so self-conscious about their bodies that they don't have time to notice yours. Find a swimming cossie you're comfortable in, and when you're walking across to the pool, think of something else, not yourself. Think about next week's physics test or the world's population explosion. Then jump in. And on the beach, remember that too much sunbathing is bad for your skin. Cover yourself in a sarong-style skirt if you really hate exposing your body. You don't have to strip off just because everyone else does. Do what you're comfortable with.

And I'm bad at sport. No one ever wants me on their team at school.

You need to make a distinction between competitive sports and exercise. The first one isn't right for everyone; the second is something we all need. If competitive sport isn't your scene, just grin and bear it. The brilliant centre-forward on the hockey pitch might also be a duffer at spelling, and might secretly admire your wonderful essays in English. Just because you're bad at sport doesn't mean you won't enjoy exercise. Find an exercise where you don't feel a fool. And a comforting thought is that some competitive sports don't actually provide effective exercise, especially if you're stuck out on a remote corner of a field, shivering, hoping the ball will come your way.

So what should I do to keep fit?

Anything from the shopping list of exercise below. The important thing is to pick one or two that you ENJOY. Exercise is not a punishment – it's fun. You should look forward to it, and you will, if you find the right one for you.

The couch potato's guide to exercise

1. Walking

This is the most natural form of exercise there is. Even a small amount helps. Even throwing away the remote control for the telly and walking over to change channels is a start. Better still, if you can walk to school rather than cadge a lift or take the bus, do so. And if the boy you fancy takes the bus, you can take the bus too, ask him out, then suggest you walk back from school together. The other plus point about walking is that you don't have to be good at it in order to benefit from it. And you don't have to take your clothes off. And it's not boring because the scenery changes all the time!

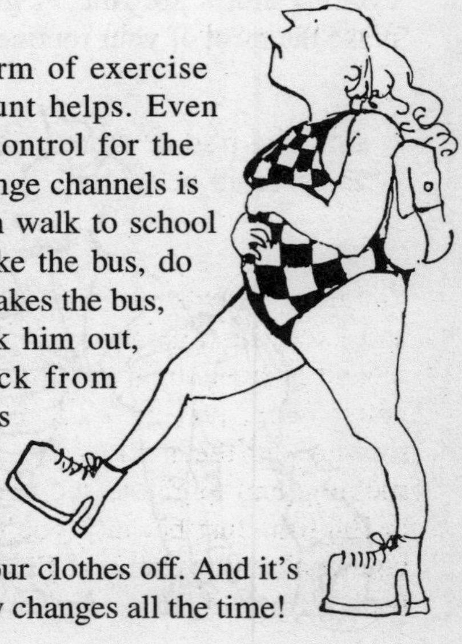

2. Swimming

Once you're actually in the water, all that's visible of you is your face, even if it's a rather wet face. Anything you do in the water, even a half-hearted doggy paddle, will do you good, as water provides resistance which will make your exercise more effective. Breast stroke gives good all round exercise, and if you can get to an aqua-fit class, you'll have great fun. It's just like playing in the bath when you were a baby. A good laugh.

3. Exercise Classes

If in your school the emphasis is on competitive sport, you might join a local exercise class. These aren't necessarily expensive. If you're loaded, you can sign on at a health club, but if you're not, check in your local library to see what's on offer. Go with a friend. You don't have to dress in skin-tight lycra if you don't want to. A baggy T-shirt and cycling shorts are fine. A good instructor will help you make the most of your routine, and give you confidence.

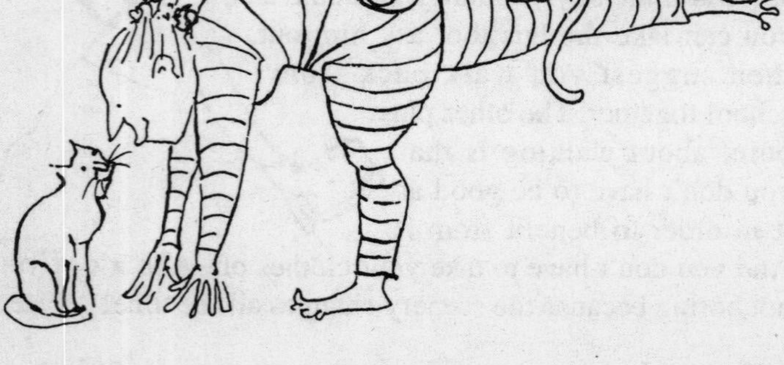

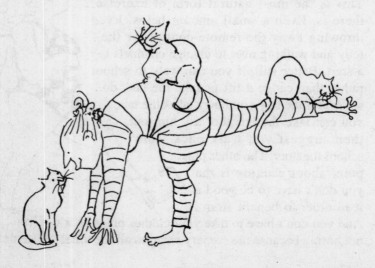

4. Exercise Videos

For the seriously self-conscious. With an exercise video you can safely exercise in the comfort of your own home. Lock the living room door in case any brothers are lurking outside, and ban the pets, as the cat is likely to come and sit on your tummy while you're doing the toning routine. Exercise videos are good for people who are short of time as you can fit them in when it suits you. But do invite your mum or a friend to check you're doing the exercises exactly like it shows on the tape, and don't be tempted to do the diet that goes with some of the exercise videos. Don't think you need to look like the glam models who lead the exercises – nobody else does, either!

5. Cycling

Provided you've got road sense, cycling regularly is another good form of keeping fit. And you can go places, too. Find a friend who cycles and do it together.

6. Dancing

Any form of dancing (except for the slow, smoochy variety) is excellent aerobic exercise. Lock yourself in your bedroom, put on something with rhythm, and go for it! Just going to a disco once a week will improve your fitness level.

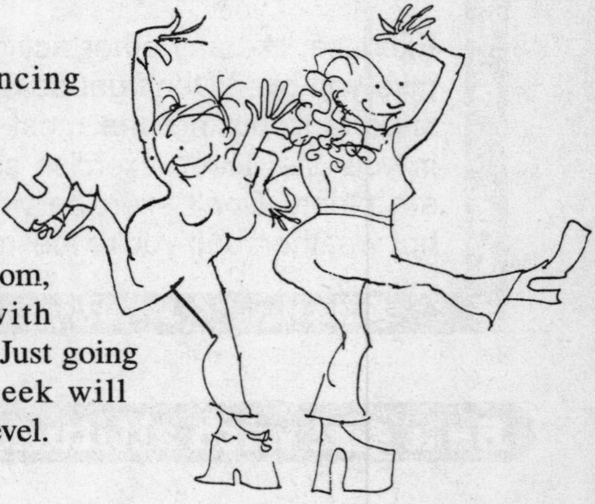

7. Skating

Take your pick – roller skating or ice skating. Provided you can keep your balance, both are great for keeping you on the move, and good for your social life, too.

8. Home Exercise Equipment

Again, it's convenient if you've got an exercise bike, or stepper or treadmill lurking at home. These can all provide you with the fitness you need. Check you know how to use them properly, and think what you'll do if they get boring. You could put your Walkman on, or even sit on the exercise bike and watch telly – as long as you remember to pedal occasionally!

Then there's jogging (always go out with someone), athletics, netball, tennis, football (yes, girls can play it too), badminton, hockey – the list is endless. Yoga is good for flexibility and relaxation, and self-defence will keep you fit. Buy yourself a pair of dead cool trainers and go for it!

... Warning ... Warning ... Warning ...

Exercise, like any other activity, ought not to take you over. Don't get obsessed with it. It's important, but not the most important thing in your life. Three exercise sessions a week are plenty. Don't exercise vigorously in very hot weather, or if you're feeling ill.

Be a girl with attitude!

Feeling good is not just about eating and exercise – but about the thoughts in your head. If you keep beating yourself up and telling yourself you're ugly, you'll end up believing yourself. Try doing the opposite.

- Stand in front of the mirror. Go on. Do it now.
- Smile at yourself. No, not just a half-hearted smirk. A real smile.
- And say these words. 'I, Ernestine, (or whatever your name is) am good-looking.'
- Have a good laugh.
- Recover from your giggles, and repeat, trying to believe it. 'I, Ernestine, am good-looking.'
- Substitute any appropriate phrase. Tell yourself you have a good figure, or lovely hair.
- Do this every day.

Another trick – get a group of your friends together and give every one a sheet of paper. Each person must write their name on the top of a sheet of paper. Then you put all the sheets of paper on a table. Everyone goes round and writes something about the person whose name is heading the paper, and this something must be something nice, and it must be true. Perhaps the person you're writing about is a very loyal friend. Say so. Write, 'You're a very loyal friend'. Or if she's brilliant at French, write that down. Or that you like her taste in clothes. Or even that you really like her. Everyone must write something on everybody else's sheet.

When you have finished, you collect the sheet with your name on the top, and read it through. This is what people really think of you. Accept it. Take the sheet of paper away with you, and stick it up in your bedroom. Read it when you're feeling low.

If you're still depressed about your appearance, and stuck in worrying about yourself, tell yourself that appearance is much less important than it seems to be. Your friends haven't chosen you, and your family doesn't love you, because of your appearance, it's because of who you really are. Have you chosen your friends because of their appearance? Probably not.

And a final exercise. When do you like yourself most? When you fit a size 10 or when you know you've been kind to someone? Worrying all the time about food and weight can make you obsessed with yourself. Take some time out to think about other people. Don't moan to your mate about your imaginary flab, but ask her how she's feeling. She'll appreciate that a lot more than you whingeing at her. Your friends like you because of the way you treat them and your mad sense of humour – not because you're thin. Wise up! And when you've got loads of mates, it's that bit easier to like yourself.

Don't get yourself into proportion, but get a sense of proportion.

In an ideal world I'd love to look like a supermodel, but I know I'm never going to. Being on the chubby side runs in our family, and I'm no exception. I'm me – I'm not going to change. I'm always hungry, and have three good meals a day. I walk to school, which is about two and a half miles. I'd never diet because all the girls I know who diet are dead boring, the way they go on about their weight. There are more interesting things in life to talk about.
(Susan, 16)

Take action

Don't just sit there – if you want to make a beginning in changing your attitude to yourself, while you're about it you can change things for others, too. Making changes is about being active, doing things.

So why don't you…

- Ask your teachers at school to provide discussion on why dieting doesn't work, and why it's self-destructive to worry too much about weight.
- Write to the magazines you read and ask them to use larger models.
- Complain to the dress shops that don't stock your size, and tell them they'd make more money if they sold larger sizes – you'd shop there, for a start.
- Write to your local newspapers if they try to recommend new diets or plaster their pages with superthin models – tell them why dieting is bad news.
- Start a group in your school to help girls with eating disorders, so they have a place to come and talk and get well again: ask a teacher to help you.
- Explain to your parents why you don't need to diet, and explain to the doctor too, if needs be.
- Be an example. Begin by not judging anyone just on their appearance. The more critical you are of other people, the more you'll imagine they're being critical of you. Think kind thoughts. Take the time to get to know people well. Then when people get to know you, they'll find out that you're worth knowing too – whatever size you are.

Chapter 11

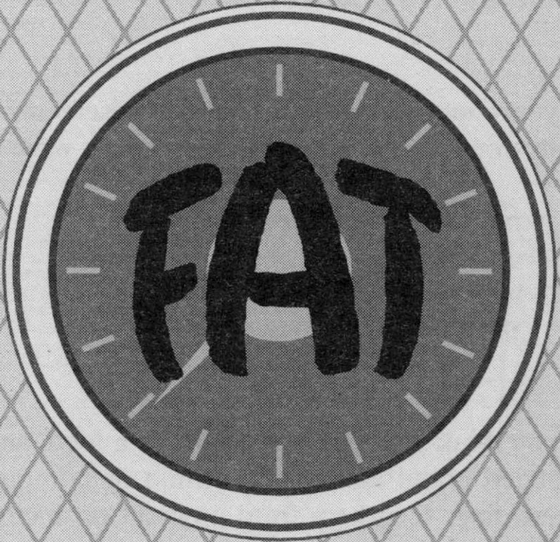

Useful information

- If you want to contact an organization that campaigns against dieting, write to...

  Mary Evans-Young,
  Dietbreakers,
  Church Cottage,
  Barford St Michael,
  Nr Deddington,
  Oxon OX15 0UA

- If you want to complain about advertisements to do with slimming or the use of thin models, write to...

  Advertising Standards Authority,
  Brook House,
  2-16 Torrington Place
  LONDON WC1E 7HN

- If you think you have a problem with food, and are worried about anorexia, bulimia or compulsive overeating, seek help from a parent or doctor. Or you can contact...

  Eating Disorders Association
  Sackville Place
  44-48 Magdalen Street
  Norwich NR3 1JU

A special helpline for 18s and under is available by ringing

01603 765050 between **4-6pm Mondays**
or **CHILDLINE 0800 1111.**

- If you want to read a glossy magazine with style tips for bigger girls, and a list of cool places to shop, try *YES!* magazine, available from WH Smith and all good newsagents.

- If you want go out on a shopping spree, try contacting the following before you set out – their youth fashions are strongly recommended.

Rogers and Rogers
Elsley House
24-30 Great Titchfield Street
LONDON W1P 7AD

Etam Plus
Jubilee House
197-213 Oxford Street
LONDON W1R 2HH

And don't overlook good ol' Marks and Sparks and Evans!